Paradoxes in Nurses' Identity, Culture and Image

This book examines some of the more disturbing representations of nurses in popular culture, to understand nursing's complex identities, challenges and future directions.

It critically analyses disquieting representations of nurses who don't care, who kill, who inspire fear or who do not comply with laws and policies. Also addressed are stories about how power is used, as well as supernatural experiences in nursing. Using a series of examples taken from popular culture ranging from film, television and novels to memoirs and true crime podcasts, it interrogates the meaning of the shadow side of nursing and the underlying paradoxes that influence professional identity. Iconic nursing figures are still powerful today. Decades after they were first created, Ratched and Annie Wilkes continue to make readers and viewers shudder at the prospect of ever being ill. Modern storytelling modes are bringing to audiences the grim reality that some nurses are members of the working poor, like Cath Hardacre in *Trust Me*, and others can be dangerous con artists, like the nurse in *Dirty John*.

This book is important reading for all those interested in understanding the links between nursing's image and the profession's potential as an agent for change.

Margaret McAllister is Professor of Nursing at Central Queensland University, Australia. With a background in nursing, mental health nursing, education and cultural studies, Margaret teaches in the Master of Mental Health Nursing and has research expertise in Narrative Therapy and Narrative Research.

Donna Lee Brien is Professor of Creative Industries at Central Queensland University, Australia. Co-editor of the *Australasian Journal of Popular Culture*, Donna's research on writing and popular culture has been widely published in scholarly and popular publications.

Routledge Research in Nursing and Midwifery

Routledge Research in Nursing and Midwifery
Pragmatic Children's Nursing
A Theory for Children and their Childhoods
Duncan C. Randall

A Theory of Cancer Care in Healthcare Settings
Edited by Carol Cox, Maya Zumstein-Shaha

Motherhood, Spirituality and Culture
Noelia Molina

Joy at Birth
An Interpretive, Hermeneutic, Phenomenological Inquiry
Susan Crowther

Paradoxes in Nurses' Identity, Culture and Image
The Shadow Side of Nursing
Margaret McAllister and Donna Lee Brien

Birthing Outside the System
The Canary in the Coal Mine
Edited by Hannah Dahlen, Bashi Kumar-Hazard and Virginia Schmied

For more information about this series, please visit: **www.routledge.com/ Routledge-Research-in-Nursing/book-series/RRIN**

Paradoxes in Nurses' Identity, Culture and Image

The Shadow Side of Nursing

Margaret McAllister and Donna Lee Brien

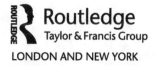
Routledge
Taylor & Francis Group

LONDON AND NEW YORK

First published 2020 by Routledge

2 Park Square, Milton Park, Abingdon, Oxon OX14 4RN
605 Third Avenue, New York, NY 10017

Routledge is an imprint of the Taylor & Francis Group, an informa business

First issued in paperback 2021

British Library Cataloguing-in-Publication Data
A catalogue record for this book is available from the British Library

Library of Congress Cataloging-in-Publication Data
A catalog record has been requested for this book

ISBN: 978-1-138-49126-7 (hbk)
ISBN: 978-1-03-217521-8 (pbk)
DOI: 10.4324/9781351033428

Typeset in Bembo
by Swales & Willis, Exeter, Devon, UK

Contents

List of figures   vi
Acknowledgements   vii

Introduction: Disquieting images of nurses   1

1   Transgressive texts about nursing   17

2   Nursing's dark past and secret knowledge   34

3   Objects of desire   51

4   Nursing and the abject   65

5   Apparitions, lost souls and healing spaces   81

6   Mighty, mean, monstrous nurses   97

7   Murdering nurses   114

8   Nurses and sick health care systems   130

9   Growing from adversity   146

Conclusion: Out of the shadows, into the light   158

Index   166

Figures

1.1 The *Getting On* team – barely tolerating each other and the demands of their work   22

3.1 A comic cartoon postcard ca. 1930s, now considered sexist and as objectifying nurses   53

4.1 Charles Dickens' fictional nurse, Sairey Gamp, embodies nursing's abject past   69

8.1 Cath Hardacre, RN a.k.a. Ally Sutton, MD – a victim or the product of a sick health care system?   132

Acknowledgements

As authors, we are indebted to the School of Nursing, Midwifery and Social Sciences and the School of Education and the Arts at Central Queensland University, Australia, for providing support and facilities for the research which has resulted in this volume. Our supervisors, Professor Moira Williamson and Professor William (Bill) Blayney have understood our commitment to this multidisciplinary project and encouraged us in its completion. A special thank you to the campus librarian, Mary Tucker, for sourcing materials at short notice.

Delegates of national and international conferences have for several years listened to our papers and provided thoughtful feedback on the research feeding into this book, and we are grateful for both those opportunities and their constructive comments. Such conferences include those of the International Health Humanities Consortium, European Society for Literature, Science and the Arts, Queensland University Educators' Showcase and the Cosmopolitanism/Women Writers/Biography symposium at the University of Queensland.

The Gothic Association of New Zealand and Australia (GANZA), Auckland University's Popular Culture Centre (and particularly their annual symposium) and the Gothic and Horror stream of the Popular Culture Association of Australian and New Zealand (PopCAANZ), all three of which are led by Associate Professor Lorna Piatti-Farnell, have been particularly generative in terms of this project. We also acknowledge Associate Professor Piatti-Farnell for helping us develop our ideas on the Gothic imaging of nurses in popular culture in the 2017 article published in the *Journal of Advanced Nursing*.

Some of this work has also been tested in publications on associated topics and themes and we thank the editors and anonymous reviewers of *Aerternum, Hecate, Journal of Advanced Nursing, Nursing Review* and *The Conversation,* for their interest in our work, and their generous and perceptive comments, which have assisted us in refining our thinking on this topic.

We would also like to thank the Noosa campus of Central Queensland University campus management and staff for their support of campus-based research events. As universities become more and more fiscally driven, many of our colleagues lack opportunities to engage collegially in the discussion of ideas that cross disciplinary boundaries and have potential to produce new theories. The *Pre-Run Re-Run* events, which we have developed and curated since 2012, have provided us with another arena for testing and refining this material, and we thank the regular attendees of these sessions for their insightful and helpful comments on work-in-progress.

Thank you to editing intern, Jo French, and to Douglas R. Atkins, Library Technician in the History of Medicine Division U.S. National Library of Medicine who assisted us in our search for permission to use the cartoon illustrating the seductive power of nurses.

A book like this takes a long time to plan, write and produce. The publishing team at Routledge have been a dream to work with. Thank you.

Finally, we thank all our colleagues, students, friends and family members who have either offered comments about, or encouragement and love during, the process of working on this book. Special and sincere thank yous to Jim, Peter Corr and Whiskey Pete (Margaret), and Wes, Kim, Kittee and Batty (Donna).

Margaret McAllister
Donna Lee Brien

Introduction

Disquieting images of nurses

A moving scene in the multiple award-winning film of Ian McEwan's (2001) novel *Atonement* (Wright, 2007), conveys a vivid image of a nurse tending to a French soldier during the Second World War. Nurse Briony Tallis quietly enters a room in which she observes a sleeping man. His head is heavily bandaged and blood seeps through the dressing. Sitting beside him, Nurse Tallis tentatively takes his hand in hers. In response to her touch, the patient awakens and begins to speak to her in a familiar way. He is obviously delirious, but the nurse maintains the conversation with him, allowing him to reminisce. In doing so, the nurse does not disavow his reality, instead she gently encourages his recall of warm croissants and consoling friendships. Feeling comforted, he then requests that the nurse loosen his bandages as he finds them too tight. Nurse Tallis complies with his wish and is visibly shaken upon seeing his horrific head wounds, but quickly composes herself to gently reapply the dressing. She remains sitting with him.

Although young and naïve, this nurse demonstrates a care that is at once compassionate and self-denying. This duality – compassion and self-denial – comprises a recognisable part of nursing's complex identity. While nurses are expected, and often motivated, to join the profession by their compassion for others (Mills, Wand and Fraser, 2015), self-denial has been noted to be a prominent aspect of nursing identity, as it was articulated and emphasised by Florence Nightingale, the influential founder of, and writer about, modern nursing in the nineteenth century. Within her vision that nursing would be both a female profession and vocation (Parker, 2005), Nightingale advocated self-sacrifice and altruism. Her vision of care was also strident, writing that

> the "new nurse" [her term for the nurses she was training] was meant to be sympathetic but detached, attentive but brisk and professional, handling any resistance on the part of the patient as if he or she was a recalcitrant child.
>
> (Nightingale, 1860)

Such a view reveals both the context in which Nightingale lived – nineteenth century Victorian England – and her middle class status at a time when nursing was a low status and dangerous task, largely performed by people (both men and women) who were old, weak, drunk and desperate (Helmstadter and Godden, 2016). Nightingale fought to raise the status of nursing to a middle-class, female profession and in the process, provided a viable career for women. As a core component of this, nurses were to be rigorously trained in order to lift standards and improve patient outcomes (Howell, 2016).

Consequently, as a result of Nightingale's leadership, for many years nursing was understood primarily in gendered and largely Victorian terms. However, as ideas about the world and health care changed, so too did thinking about nursing. Humanistic philosophies, developed from the rise of psychology in the early parts of the twentieth century, began to be applied to nursing, and values such as empathy, acceptance and person-centredness came to be seen as central to nursing identity (Peplau, 1952). This change also brought with it the possibility that nursing could be understood in human, rather than gendered terms (Parker, 2005) – illustrating two important points about identity generally: it can evolve, *but* vestiges of the past can linger in how identity is understood. The nineteenth century feminine ideal of self-sacrifice is a good example in relation to nursing identity. Although it has long been outdated in terms of contemporary nursing practice, it is still a common image of nursing in representations of the profession in the media and popular culture. As well as an exemplar of humanity, Nurse Tallis is also pretty, slender, gentle, genteel and extremely feminine in appearance and all her actions. In her white uniform and pert cap, she is the embodiment of a stereotype that many would imagine when asked to visualise a nurse. Such images are common in the media and in popular culture, as are many others that use the image of nurses and nursing to represent and, at times, disparage women. While these images have been criticised as denigrating nurses and nursing by those within the profession (Darbyshire, 2010; Ferns and Chojnacka, 2005), this book suggests that such representational practices are also extremely revealing and, as such, worthy of sustained consideration and analysis. Such an analysis is important not only as this imagery affects the way contemporary nursing is understood by others outside the profession, but also how nurses understand themselves. This self-understanding reflects upon, and influences, nursing's own culture and history, including its challenges. These challenges involve struggles with personal, institutional and systemic manifestations of power, hierarchy and control, and how these can be understood and addressed.

Looking closely at how nurses and nursing are represented is also of value and, as this book proposes, nursing is also an important social artefact – its position and value within communities operates like a social barometer. This can be seen when negative actions and issues are exposed in the media or portrayed in popular culture – what could be described as "nurses behaving badly" – for such incidents are frequently an indicator of more deeply seated social, economic or cultural problems. For example, "undemure" protests by nurses, involving strike actions that can be criticised as putting patients at risk

(Clarke and O'Neill, 2001) are often in relation to trying to secure better patient-nurse ratios when governments apply austerity policies and tighten health budgets. Some media stories of "bad nursing" are similarly sometimes simply the result of impossible workloads.

There are also disturbing and complex issues that afflict the culture of nursing, but which remain hidden in the shadows. These are the dark, more obscure and sometimes even sinister aspects of nursing that are covered up and hidden from view in health care practice, discourse and policy-making, either deliberately or unintentionally. These issues are, however, often represented in popular culture narratives – in films, television series, popular novels and other forms. When identified and analysed, these less obvious features of the profession offer fascinating insights into nurses and nursing. In doing so, such an investigation possesses the potential to advance a more nuanced understanding of nursing's complex history, identity, challenges and future directions.

Nurses and nursing today

Nurses play such a recognised role in society that children as young as three are aware of them (Archer, 1984), with much of this knowledge coming from their representation in popular culture. Nursing has been in existence for thousands of years, with the earliest manifestations in India, around the first century BC (Svoboda, 1992), but the representation of nursing within popular culture and the mass media do not necessarily broadcast a realistic image of nursing's past or present. This is significant because the public gains an unrealistic idea of the reality of what to expect from nursing care from such sources, and nurses and those seeking to join the profession in the future are given idealistic and simplified ideas about the work that ultimately glosses over the complexities of this profession. For both the public and nursing profession, the imaging of nurses in popular culture ignores and, even worse, dismisses serious problems that need to be tackled and resolved. As this volume will describe, despite nurses being embedded within communities as healers for thousands of years, it is only relatively recently that nursing became gendered, giving rise to a paternalist and mystical discourse that has confined and patronised nurses as a group. This gendering simplifies the challenges that affect nurses and nursing, while also feeding into anxieties felt by the public when they feel let down by the health system, or when their unspoken needs are not met by a supposedly all-knowing, ever-present nurse.

The trouble with this repeated and unreflective imaging of nurses in popular culture and the media is that such representations have taken on a fixed and mythic status, from where they inform but also mislead and misdirect, in the process feeding into both wishful thinking and cultural anxieties. For example, images of nurses as nurturing mother figures and gentle ministering angels (like Nurse Tallis) have been very effective in highlighting the valuable work that nursing provides, particularly in times of crises like war and other catastrophes. Such good press can, of course, be flattering for nurses, whose work might otherwise go unnoticed and unappreciated. But this representation is also unrealistic and dehumanising, for nurses are neither mothers nor celestial beings, and thus ironically, they are being set up to fail – both the public and themselves. The book does not argue that this imaging of nurses and nursing in the mass media and popular culture should not exist. Indeed, this example of *Atonement* and many others discussed are highly entertaining, creative and, at times, major works of considerable artistic merit. Others have no claims to be anything else but popular entertainment, and this motivation – or effect – is not problematised in this discussion. Rather, this book works from the existence of this plethora of representation, to argue that this imaging needs to be more closely surveyed and analysed.

The shadow side of nursing

Conversely, many scholars of nursing have decried what they perceive as the damage caused by such stereotyping. There are even organisations that check and criticise media producers who promulgate what they judge to be sexist or demeaning stories about nurses (as, for example, the American not-for-profit organisation, The Truth About Nursing, 2019). There are, however, downsides to this control over how nursing can be spoken about, including that much about the profession is sanitised, and its complexity is erased. Darker narratives that subvert the ideal of the self-sacrificing, ever-caring nurse successfully offering healing succour are largely not addressed, and thus remain untheorised. Consequently, scholars, the public and nurses themselves have a limited lexicon with which to describe a large part of the reality of nursing work, which is situated in the realm of the abject and profane, the turbulent and traumatic. Similarly, many find it difficult, even impossible, to understand how good nurses may turn away from their oath to protect those in their care, going so far as to even maim and kill, or why nurses with a detailed knowledge of health disregard what they know to be healing and helpful.

Even less is known about the subjective and embodied ways of being, thinking and acting that are at the heart of many nursing rituals and private discussions – overshadowed as they are by the more objective, credible and dominant discourses of logical-rationalism and scientific evidence-based practice. Nursing conversations on night shift, for instance, frequently venture into the shadows, as nurses exchange supposedly true stories of *déjà vu* and near-death experiences, and ghost stories that defy logical explanation. This discourse is often dismissed as vernacular and peripheral, but it is also replete with meaning for, and about, nurses and nursing culture. In this way, black comedy or even more transgressive texts that show nurses acting uncharacteristically and transcending the normal constraints placed upon expected nursing behaviours, can also be informative.

Instead of shying away from such texts, analysis of them suggests that even the most disquieting representations of "bad" nurses and nursing (McAllister and Brien, 2016a) are vital for nurses' professional understanding and broader cultural memory. A quintessential story of corruption and evil is found, for instance, in the Nazi nurses of the Second World War (Benedict and Shields, 2014), a subject that is little discussed but that is just beginning to be a fertile subject for film and other media narratives. Like these examples, there are many other nurses who appear to embody the direct opposite of a caring persona. These include nurses who are serial killers (Graeber, 2014) or mercy killers (Fink, 2009), as well as those who have misled and caused harm in unethical medical experiments (Smith, 1996), engaged in other anti-social acts (Field, 2007; McAllister and Brien, 2016a, 2016b) and/or not complied with the overarching laws and policies that should have guided their practice (Hutchinson, 1992; Jackson et al., 2010; Lamb et al., 2017). Fictional representations, including in the genres of horror, crime, parody and pornography, make heavy use of nurses acting subversively (McAllister, Brien and Piatti-Farnell, 2017), and are – in this context – useful to consider.

Many nurses also work in areas of care that are considered taboo or barbaric – on death row, or in detention centres and refugee camps, for example. Many work closely with people who are marginalised, stigmatised or harshly judged by society at large – people with mental disorders, and the aging, addicted, or those afflicted with contagious diseases, for instance. Ignoring the realities of this work can further marginalise and deny the patients who depend on that care, and also those who choose to deliver it. In addition, this lack of acknowledgment can severely impact the productivity and sustainability of a profession which suffers from significant attrition. As the largest profession in health care world-wide, nursing also has the highest turnover rate (Duffield et al., 2014). The stressful nature of the work, its fast pace, high-stakes, and increasingly complex treatments and technologies, paired with the threat of job insecurity and low pay, are fuelling widespread disenchantment with nursing as a career and fuelling ever-growing numbers reporting an intention to leave the profession (Traynor, 2017).

Many nurses have also found, or find, themselves in a range of abject situations: witnessing misery, pain, torture, death or slow and painful human decline. In delivering routine health care, nurses regularly encounter anxiety, fear, sorrow, anger and even violence. They come in intimate contact with – smelling, seeing and touching – wounds that bleed and leak. They deal with bodily decay and excreta. This association with the abject constitutes a familiar, but often unspoken, dark side of nursing's everyday work (Rudge and Holmes, 2010).

Nurses are also permitted to transgress numerous personal and human boundaries. They access patients' bodies in extremely intimate ways, and they are privy to intensely personal thoughts, feelings and confessions. They are also immersed in the same feelings and tensions that can overwhelm patients, such as fear, anxiety, fatigue and helplessness. This is not an easy way of working, or of being. Yet airing and discussing such dark – and again, largely silenced – complexities may render them less repellent and more understandable (Lawler, 2006).

Within education studies, an emerging body of work explores what is known as "negative capability" (Saggurthi and Thakur, 2016). Negative capability involves imaginatively and concertedly staying in the realm of "not knowing", and considering those aspects of life that involve uncertainty, mystery, doubt or anxiety. This means checking the automatic desire to speedily control a problem with a quick-fix or pragmatic solution in order to come to a higher level and more viable approach to care (Rushmer and Davies, 2004). Yet, temporary and simplistic approaches are characteristic of health care management regimes that celebrate action (French, Simpson and Harvey, 2009) and decisive activity. The value placed on being fast and definitive, however, leads to the avoidance of difficult questions and the denial of human failings and frailties (Saggurthi and Thakur, 2016). It is a reality, for example, that all nurses (and doctors and other health care workers) sometimes make mistakes and formulate limited and faulty diagnoses and will continue to do so. There is also a growing awareness that nursing as a profession, while nurses are themselves growing in numbers and skill level, is deeply hampered by unresolved problems (Lakeman and Molloy, 2018).

Considering such challenging, negative and even taboo aspects of nursing can help generate awareness and new knowledge that may help transform a culture of upheaval and dissatisfaction into one that flourishes and thrives. As this seems so difficult to achieve in practice, looking to media representations is, this volume suggests, one way to begin. This draws on an interdisciplinary analysis, in order to produce novel information to feed into finding solutions to such seemingly intractable problems (McAllister and Brien, 2016a).

Storytelling has been the prominent way that humans communicate and share their culture with each other. Storytelling has long been a part of nursing's culture (Wolf, 2008), and more recently it has been enjoying a resurgence (Le Blanc, 2017; Timbrell, 2017; Wadsworth, 2017). Yet, many of the stories being told in nursing are what Frank (1998) describes as restitution narratives. Like much traditional crime fiction, where the criminal is identified and brought to justice by the end of the story (Knight, 2010), restitution narratives convey the notion that tension and conflict have been resolved and, in doing so, they simplify or overlook the complexities, ongoing oppositions and paradoxes that may underlie the plot or characterisations in the story. This ultimately preserves prevailing cultural ideologies, leaving them unchallenged and the status quo maintained. This book seeks to uncover and analyse a series of more complex narratives about nurses and nursing in order to identify and problematise this dominant discourse.

Many stories about nursing have been criticised for perpetuating stereotypes. As we discuss in the following chapters, common stereotypes include the angel of mercy, the hand-maiden and the battleaxe. However, the literature on these commonly used and widely recognised stereotypes rarely explores the origin of these stereotypes. Nor does it consider them as conveying archetypal stories that may contain morals and deep meaning. In seeking to look into and beyond stereotypes, this book focuses on stories of nursing's dark side – something that Jung referred to as a "shadow side".

According to Jung (1969), human beings are not born as a blank slate. Rather, they have written within them instincts and archetypes that have been transmitted inter-generationally through family or religious groups, and through humankind. Jung described archetypal events that have universal meaning. These include the rites of birth, death, separation from parents, initiations and marriage that seem to occur in every cultural group across the ages. He also described archetypal figures, such as the mother, father, child, god, devil, trickster and hero figures that occur – and recur – in many myths and stories. In addition, he also identified archetypal motifs, such as the creation, the deluge and the apocalypse that are all deeply meaningful across cultures. The shadow was one of Jung's archetypical motifs. He also believed that these archetypes can only be viewed indirectly – through myths, stories, artworks, or dreams – and that, when they are examined, and their morals internalised, they can help to balance and integrate the unconscious with the conscious, and to transform the self.

Jung considered that the human being is complex, with a personality that is made up of that which is consciously projected – our persona, which is what we would like others to see – and a hidden, opposite side to our self which is repressed into the unconscious. Jung referred to this as "the shadow" because it consists of primitive, negative or socially disparaged emotions like lust, anger and shame. This part of the personality is "dark" and unenlightened because it is completely obscured from consciousness. Yet it is also an ever-present shadow, connected to the self, influencing behaviour and contributing to the whole. In Jung's words, "everyone carries a shadow, and the less it is embodied in the individual's conscious life, the blacker and denser it is" (1938, p. 131). As Jungian analysts explain, negative proclivities, which we all have, tend to be repressed as shadow archetypes, stored within the collective unconscious, and projected onto unwitting adversaries. Unfortunately, all too frequently, there are reports of this occurring in health care, with nurses projecting their own unprocessed anxieties. This manifests in various ways: as lateral violence directed towards other nurses (Roberts, 2015); as patients bearing the brunt of stress and being neglected or dehumanised (Haque and Waytz, 2012); and when doctors are disparaged and unfairly criticised by nurses (Fagin and Garelick, 2004).

Nurses' professional identity

Having a sense of one's identity involves having a sense of oneself that provides a source of motivation, self-efficacy and satisfaction (Gecas, 2000).

Individual and more collective identity also evolves over time, as worldly experiences, relationships and knowledge grow and are incorporated into understanding (Harter, 1997). When an individual develops a clear sense of their own identity, they appreciate their uniqueness as well as their connectedness or difference from others, and are able to function in the social world with confidence. This is also applicable to professional and other forms of collective identity.

Identity can also be positively or negatively shaped by peer, cultural and social values (Cote and Levine, 2014). The same is true for an individual's professional identity. Like a child, a novice nurse begins their career with no clear identity and relies on parental, external figures and role models like educators and expert nurses to tell them what to believe and how to behave. As that new nurse develops a professional persona through their experiences and in their relationships with others, their professional identity may begin to change. They may discard beliefs and values that are not a good fit, and take up others that feel more in keeping with the group with which they identify (Tyler, Kramer and John, 2014). Ultimately, and ideally, a professional identity allows an individual to know who they are and what they stand for, and supports them in sourcing their values and beliefs from within. A strong professional identity provides a clear sense of purpose, strengthens commitment and provides direction for the future. Without such clarity, confusion, doubt, dissatisfaction and identity diffusion can occur (Schott, Van Kleef and Noordegraaf, 2016). As a nurse develops from neophyte to confident practitioner, their exposure to external sources that convey beliefs about nursing may be influential. If those sources are negative, outdated, constrictive or unrealistic, and are accepted uncritically, identity may become distorted, stunted or maladapted. Therefore, it is important for nurses to be able to identify and process external representations of, and beliefs about, nurses and nursing, in order that their sense of a professional identity is strengthened by such informed knowledge.

The good nurse

If there is a grand narrative circulating in popular culture, and society itself, about nursing and nursing identity, it is the idea of "the good nurse". The personification of this image is, of course, Florence Nightingale, who famously described and documented the attributes of a good nurse. In 1881, she wrote in a letter to nurses at St Thomas' Hospital in London, that "to be a good nurse one must be a good woman . . . What makes a good woman is the better or higher of their nature: Quietness, Gentleness, Patience, Endurance, Forbearance" (collected in Vicinus and Nergaard 1989, 385). This nineteenth century image of perfect womanhood included other attributes that were seen then as attractive feminine qualities in the domestic sphere, such as being demure, compliant, composed and self-abrogating. This notion was so prevalent at this time that such women became characterised as "the angel in the house" (Patmore, 1866). Nightingale appropriated this ideal for nursing to image her nurses as angels in hospitals. Many aspects of this good woman/ good nurse have persisted in current imagination, and contribute to stereotypes of the nurse today. This is despite the radical social, cultural, technological and bio-medical reforms in the last 150 years, not least of which has been a considerable increase in the number of male nurses. Not only has Nightingale herself become a powerful symbol of nursing, the ideas she espoused have been, and continue to be, reproduced across a wide range of media, including novels, music, poetry and film.

The brief, but highly evocative, portrayal of Nurse Tallis in *Atonement* described at the opening of this chapter draws upon these embedded beliefs about the attributes and behaviours of a good nurse. Nurse Tallis is caring, composed, gentle, fair, pretty, clean, tidy and feminine; she is also obedient and compliant. She uses a range of skills to provide comfort to her patient, and is not too busy to provide highly personalised and sensitive human contact in order to meet her patient's needs.

Nelson and Gordon (2006) argue that the trope of the good nurse simplifies and obscures the complexity of contemporary nursing. In reality, individual nurses often act in ways that defy this notion, but the idea of the good nurse is so prevalent that it is widely accepted not only by patients but within nursing itself and so, when nurses fail to live up to the stereotype, they are sanctioned. Nelson and Gordon's criticism of the deficiencies of the good nurse trope can be applied to the *Atonement* story. This is because the gentle caregiving that Nurse Tallis embodies – although undoubtedly accepted and valorised in the early twentieth century and promulgated in numerous stories about that era as, for instance, *Anzac Girls* (ABC, 2014) and *Crimson Field* (BBC, 2014) – is not the sum of nursing skills needed in contemporary health care. Although the novelist and film makers may have intended for the readers and audience to view Nurse Tallis as a woman of a certain time and place, the beauty and power of the narrative makes her character timeless. Using the good nurse trope in this story makes her, as a character, not only potently familiar, but also highly attractive. However, hers is a characterisation that is also subtly loaded with a narrow view of women's work and nursing's challenges. At the very least, *Atonement* portrays nursing in a highly romantic way that is limiting. Routine practices are not the same today as they were in the past and nor are interpersonal relationships. Nurses cannot be demure when they are expected to take responsibility. They cannot be emotional when they need to be impartial decision makers. They also cannot risk placing themselves in clinical situations that are beyond their competence.

This means that contemporary nurses – and the profession of nursing more broadly – have to acknowledge and actively break away from the stereotype of the good nurse. To accomplish this, nurses need to be aware of where it comes from, why it exists and how it continues to operate. They also need to be prepared to reflect on how it may have been unconsciously adopted despite being so unhelpful in contemporary practice. Nurse Tallis, for example, displays tremendous fortitude and a deep ethic of humanity and care, but her silent obedience is not a quality that is useful for contemporary nurses. Her character reveals a paradox about the good nurse in the contemporary world. The universal and timeless values of kindness and compassion that she displays remain appealing, but it is doubtful she would possess the toughness and resilience necessary to withstand the harsh realities of modern nursing. This reveals an impossible inconsistency at the heart of the good nurse trope. On one hand, the image is very complementary to nurses, and enormously validating. The image acknowledges a nurse's value, wisdom, creativity, selflessness, integrity and valour. However, by repeatedly constructing nurses as good, angelic or in other related one-dimensional and unrealistic ways, nurses are effectively dehumanised and undermined. For nurses are not perfect, ever-virtuous angels. They are human beings and as such, capable of making mistakes, and of reaching their psychological and physical limits.

While many of Nightingale's aspirations for nursing are positive, the net effect of this pervasive stereotyping of the nurse is to sentimentalise and trivialise what is, in fact, the highly skilled work of nursing. This means there is also a mismatch between many ongoing fictional representations of nurses and the contemporary realities of nursing. This book explores this and other paradoxes, by analysing the full range of representations of nurses – from the perfect to the monstrous – in order unpack the culture, history and challenges facing nursing in a way that illuminates new possibilities for nursing's identity and image (Roberts, 2000). Such an analysis would suggest that, despite the serenely beautiful and ultimately profoundly moving portrayal of Nurse Tallis in *Atonement* and her humane actions with the dying soldier, her compliance with the notion of what counts for good nursing locks her into a role that is limiting for her. In embodying the good nurse stereotype, she cannot, for instance, utilise her personal potential power at the social and political level, protesting for instance, her part in the war machine.

Imagery itself can be paradoxical, as in how nurses in popular culture can be simultaneously revered and feared. A clear example is the battleaxe matron, a stereotype within popular culture that links the display of female power with alarm and destruction (see, Darbyshire and Gordon, 2005). This depiction parallels the ambivalent way that female leaders of all kinds are portrayed within contemporary culture and is itself deserving of close analysis.

Popular culture and mass media

Although relatively underexplored in scholarship, this book follows suggestions that there is a dark side to nursing – the individual actions of nurses – that should be more widely and fully discussed (see, for instance, Darbyshire, 2018). Given the pervasiveness of the good nurse trope, it is not easy to explore negative and even gruesome aspects of nursing in practice, but this dimension is readily accessible through its representations in popular culture and in the media. Hence, this book draws upon numerous examples of such

texts to explore images of nursing and the paradoxical ways such representations both reflects, and influences, nurses and society. Using a wide selection
of texts, we reveal and interpret the problematic, paradoxical or ironic. Many
genres are used, including works of comedy, memoir and documentary,
alongside horror or drama. Dominant ideas can seep into culture so deeply
that they become naturalised, taken-for-granted and no longer noticed or
contested. But revealing and interrogating these ideologies and myths can
lead to a fuller understanding of how, in this case, realities of nursing practice
differ from projected ideas and ideals, and what this might mean for nursing's
identity and position within the world.

Culture is the medium by which social structures maintain themselves
(Giroux, 2000). Popular culture is said to be "the bricks and mortar of our
most commonplace understandings", because "it is one of the fundamental
paradoxes of our social life that when we are at our most natural, our most
everyday, we are also at our most cultural" (Willis, 1979, pp. 184–185).
Selected films, television programmes, novels and news stories provide a rich
vein of material about nurses and nursing, as do less conventional sources
such as memoirs, poetry, works of art, music, photographs, museum and art
exhibitions and online sources, such as blogs. In exploring a series of counter-narratives to that of the good nurse, the following chapters take
a thematic approach to both a series of deeply serious and often troubling
stories and behaviours, as well as others that can be classed as more gently
entertaining, mockingly carnivalesque (Bakhtin, 1929, 1941) or dangerously
trivialising. This is, in itself, an interesting paradox, because it appears that the
more nursing's image is broadcast, and the more visible the profession
becomes, this prominence also suppresses and obscures nursing's social and
political position within society.

Chapter 1 explores the notion of transgressive texts, and in this specific
context, where the good nurse trope is subverted or replaced. We examine
how these transgressive texts offer a way of casting light on anxieties that are
often largely unspoken and unrecognised within mainstream culture. These
include that nurses may display human inconsistencies and frailties and that
the health care system may itself be flawed.

Chapter 2 discusses nursing's dark past when, rather than science and evidence-based practice holding sway, nurses drew upon a knowledge of the
"healing arts" that was passed down from elder to novice. We discuss how
nurses continue to value the arts-based part of their work although this can,
paradoxically, put them at risk of being viewed with suspicion. Yet this curi-
ous position is also what helps to make nursing characters in popular culture
so compelling.

In Chapter 3, an unseemly side of nursing – the nurse as a sex object – is
examined. The sexualisation of nursing's image is long standing and contributes significantly to the public discourse about nurses. While considering the
negative impact on nursing of this objectification, the chapter also explores
what the ongoing desire for intimacy with a nurse means when read using

psychoanalytic theory and the nature of repression and projection. We explore how the associations of desirability, fondness and familiarity that feed into the idea of nurses as "sexy" are positive in terms of the public's view of nursing and, thus, it may be possible for these aspects to strengthen nursing's identity and place within the social world.

Staying firmly within this darker side of nursing, Chapter 4 considers those aspects of the professional role that are disgusting, and which require nurses to possess coping strategies that allow them to suppress natural responses and get the task completed. In managing the abject in this way, nursing work involves highly developed self-control that simultaneously eases a patient's concerns and fosters respect. So, in this examination of the profane, some of what is sacred and admired about nursing becomes apparent.

Chapter 5 continues this discussion of the sacred by exploring the spiritual and religious roots of nursing and how this heritage continues to influence the thoughts, values and practices of some nurses today. Acknowledgement of the presence of spirit – be it in the life-force that keeps dying patients alive, or the factor that ensures nurses retain an irrepressible buoyancy even in the face of setbacks – provides an important counterpoint to a health care world that is growing increasingly clinical and cold. A belief in the supernatural is contrasted with the reliance on the techno-scientific in nursing practice and training.

Chapter 6 focuses on the many nurses in popular culture who quintessentially embody the notion of the monstrous. From battleaxes to the domineering, to those grotesque, manipulative psychopaths hell-bent on revenge and murder, many – although not all – of these fictional characters are women. This chapter considers what this compelling negative imagining of the nurse means in terms of the working nurse's image and identity.

Chapter 7 furthers a focus on the terrifying figure of the murderous nurse, but concentrating instead on this representation in popular non-fiction narratives. Beginning with the example of the darkest hour of nursing's history, nurses' participation in the Nazi eugenics programme during the Second World War, the chapter then explores other cases of people who made a conscious decision to become a nurse in order to hurt and exploit others. The chapter outlines the lessons nursing can learn from these stories, including that nurses cannot simply be bystanders when what is happening is wrong or corruption is evident.

Chapter 8 examines stories about dysfunctional health care systems, both fictional and those based on real events, and the nurses who worked in them, either participating in the chaos, or fighting to correct injustice as whistle-blowers. It is acknowledged that nursing is a role that requires courage to stand up for what is right.

Chapter 9 showcases the stories of nurses who inspire hope and change. Although nursing is stressful because nurses witness patient distress and suffering daily, there are numerous accounts where they have faced adversity with courage and resilience. Stories where nurses step out of the shadows are as revealing as they are inspirational.

The Conclusion traces the thematic threads that have emerged in this investigation of the shadow side of nursing: the anxieties, paradoxes and aspects of nursing identity that such transgressive representations reveal.

Conclusion

Currently, both nursing and nursing's problems are in the shadows. This volume argues that nursing remains a mystery to the public – and, largely, to nurses – because nurses often stand in the long shadow cast by modern medicine. Like Freud's use of the metaphor "the dark continent" (2002) to describe what he thought was the inscrutability of women, much of nursing's way of being and working is hidden and remains unknown and untheorised. If the identities of individual nurses and nursing as a profession are to strengthen, and health care is to improve, then nursing must examine its vulnerabilities, problems and professional obstacles. Without exploring and theorising nurses, their work and the nurse's way of being in the world, it is not possible to speak about nursing coherently and completely, to revise and research the practices within it, or to provide possible pathways to solutions for currently intractable problems.

This book, therefore, examines the hidden sides of nursing via the vehicle of its representations in popular culture and the media, in the process offering a new lexicon for articulating ideas about nursing. This, we believe, enlarges the vocabulary available to articulate the profession's complexity and how current challenges might be met. This approach opens up discussion regarding situations and actions that have heretofore been too embarrassing, shameful, perplexing or counter-intuitive to address or that, when broached, have been impossible to express, let alone comprehend. Without open and frank discussion, such issues remain buried and, when they are exposed, become traumatic and stressful. Yet, when brought into the light and interrogated, these same issues can become the basis for cautionary tales. Such admonitions offer a way for those with a vested interest – such as current or future nurses, as well as those who lead, educate or legislate about them, for example – to harness and mobilise effective resistance, resilience and change strategies.

References

Archer C (1984) Children's attitudes towards sex-role division in adult occupational roles *Sex Roles* 10(1/2): 1–10.

Bakhtin M (1929) *Problems of Dostoevsky's Poetics*. Minneapolis: University of Minnesota Press.

Bakhtin M (1941) *Rabelais and His World*. Bloomington: Indiana University Press.

Benedict S and Shields L (2014) *Nurses and Midwives in Nazi Germany: The "Euthanasia Programs"*. New York: Routledge, Taylor & Francis Group.

Carneron K and Watson I (2014) *Anzac Girls*. Sydney: Screentime Productions.

Clark R, Evans D and O'Sullivan T (2014) *Crimson Field*. London: BBC Productions.

Clarke J and O'Neill C (2001) An analysis of how the *Irish Times* portrayed Irish nursing during the 1999 strike *Nursing Ethics* 8(4): 350–359.

Cote J E and Levine C G (2014) *Identity, Formation, Agency, and Culture: A Social Psychological Synthesis*. Hove: Psychology Press.

Darbyshire P (2010) Heroines, hookers and harridans: Exploring popular images and representations of nurses and nursing. In Daly J, Speedy S and Jackson D (eds) *Contexts of Nursing*. Chatswood: Elsevier, 51–64.

Darbyshire P (2018) Nursing a media grievance *Journal of Clinical Nursing* 27(7–8): e1242–e1243.

Darbyshire P and Gordon S (2005) Exploring popular images and representations of nurses and nursing. In Daly J, Speedy S, Jackson D, Lambert V and Lambert C (eds) *Professional Nursing: Concepts, Issues, and Challenges*. New York: Springer, 69–92.

Duffield C M, Roche M A, Homer C, Buchan J and Dimitrelis S (2014) A comparative review of nurse turnover rates and costs across countries. *Journal of Advanced Nursing* 70(12): 2703–2712.

Fagin L and Garelick A (2004) The doctor-nurse relationship *Advances in Psychiatric Treatment* 10(4): 277–286.

Ferns T and Chojnacka I (2005) Angels and swingers, matrons and sinners: Nursing stereotypes *British Journal of Nursing* 14(19): 1028–1032.

Field J (2007) *Caring to Death: A Discursive Analysis of Nurses Who Murder Patients*. PhD Thesis. Adelaide: University of Adelaide.

Fink S (2009) The deadly choices at Memorial. *New York Times Magazine* 30: 28–46.

Frank A W (1998) Just listening: Narrative and deep illness. *Families, Systems, & Health*, 16(3): 197.

French R, Simpson P and Harvey C (2009) Negative capability: A contribution to the understanding of creative leadership. In *Psychoanalytic Studies of Organizations: Contributions from the International Society for the Psychoanalytic Study of Organizations*. London: Karnac, 197–216.

Freud S (2002) *Wild Analysis*. Translated by Alan Bance with an Introduction by Adam Phillips. London: Penguin.

Gecas V (2000) Value identities, self-motives, and social movements. *Self, Identity, and Social Movements* 13: 93–109.

Giroux H (2000) *Impure Acts: The Practical Politics of Cultural Studies*. New York: Routledge.

Graeber C (2014) *The Good Nurse: A True Story of Medicine, Madness and Murder*. New York: Hachete Book Group.

Haque O S and Waytz A (2012) Dehumanization in medicine: Causes, solutions, and functions. *Perspectives on Psychological Science* 7(2): 176–186.

Harter S (1997) The personal self in social context. *Self and Identity: Fundamental Issues* 1: 81–105.

Helmstadter C and Godden J (2016) *Nursing before Nightingale, 1815–1899*. London: Routledge.

Howell J (2016) Nurse going native: Language and identity in letters from Africa and the British West Indies. *The Journal of Commonwealth Literature* 51(1): 165–181.

Hutchinson S (1992) Nurses who violate the Nurse Practice Act: Transformation of professional identity. *Journal of Nursing Scholarship* 24(2): 133–140.

Jackson D, Peters K, Andrew S, Edenborough M, Halcomb E, Luck L, Salamonson Y and Wilkes L (2010) Understanding whistleblowing: Qualitative insights from nurse whistleblowers. *Journal of Advanced Nursing* 66(10): 2194–2201.

Jung C G (1938) Psychology and religion. In CW 11: *Psychology and Religion: West and East*. London: Pantheon, 131.

Jung C G (1953) *Two Essays on Analytical Psychology*. London: Princeton University Press, 277.

Jung C G (1969) *Archetypes and the Collective Unconscious. Collected Works of C.G. Jung. Volume 9 (Part 1)*. Princeton: Princeton University Press.

Knight S (2010) *Crime Fiction since 1800: Detection, Death, Diversity*. London: Macmillan International Higher Education.

Lakeman R and Molloy L (2018) Rise of the zombie institution, the failure of mental health nursing leadership, and mental health nursing as a zombie category. *International Journal of Mental Health Nursing* 27(3): 1009–1014.

Lamb M, Babenko-Mould Y, Wong C and Kirkwood K (2017) Conscience, conscientious objection, and nursing: A concept analysis. *Journal of Nursing Ethics* 26(1): 37–49.

Lawler J (2006) *Behind the Screens: Nursing, Somology, and the Problem of the Body*. Sydney: Sydney University Press.

LeBlanc R (2017) Digital story telling in social justice nursing education. *Public Health Nursing* 34(4), 395–400.

McAllister M and Brien D L (2016a) Narratives of the "not-so-good nurse": Rewriting nursing's virtue script. *Hecate* 41(1/2): 79–97.

McAllister M and Brien D L (2016b) Psychiatric museums: The return of the undead asylum. *Aeternum: The Journal of Contemporary Gothic Studies* 3(1): 49–62.

McAllister M, Brien D L and Piatti-Farnell L (2017) Tainted love: Gothic imaging of nurses in popular culture. *Journal of Advanced Nursing* 74(2): 310–317.

McEwan I (2001) *Atonement*. London: Random House.

Mills J, Wand T and Fraser J A (2015) On self-compassion and self-care in nursing: Selfish or essential for compassionate care? *International Journal of Nursing Studies* 52: 791–793.

Nelson S and Gordon S (eds) (2006) *The Complexities of Care: Nursing Reconsidered*. New York: ILR Press.

Nightingale F (1860) *Notes on Nursing: What It Is and What It Is Not*. London: Harrison.

Nightingale, F (1881) Letter to the nurses and probationers of St Thomas' Hospital, London, 6 May. In Vicinus M and Nergaard B (eds). *Ever Yours, Florence Nightingale: Selected Letters*. Cambridge: Harvard University Press, 385–386.

Parker J (2005) Nursing identity and difference. *Nursing Inquiry* 12(2): 65.

Patmore C (1866) *The Angel in the House*. London: Macmillan.

Peplau H E (1952) Interpersonal relations in nursing. *The American Journal of Nursing* 52(6): 765.

Roberts S J (2000) Development of a positive professional identity: Liberating oneself from the oppressor within. *Advances in Nursing Science* 22(4): 71–82.

Roberts S J (2015) Lateral violence in nursing: A review of the past three decades. *Nursing Science Quarterly* 28(1): 36–41.

Rudge T and Holmes D eds (2010) *Abjectly Boundless*. Surrey: Ashgate Publishing.

Rushmer R and Davies H (2004) Unlearning in health care. *British Medical Journal, Quality & Safety*. 13(Supp 2): ii10–ii15.

Saggurthi S and Thakur M (2016) Usefulness of uselessness: A case for negative capability in management. *Academic Management and Learning Education* 15(1): 180–193.

Schott C, Van Kleef D and Noordegraaf M (2016) Confused professionals?: Capacities to cope with pressures on professional work. *Public Management Review* 18(4): 583–610.

Smith S (1996) Neither victim nor villain: Nurse Eunice Rivers, the Tuskegee syphilis experiment, and public health work. *Journal of Womens' History* 8(1): 95–113.

Svoboda R (1992) *Ayurveda: Life, Health and Longevity*. London: Penguin Books.

The Truth About Nursing (2019) Available at: https://thetruthaboutnursing.org.

Timbrell, J. (2017) Instructional storytelling: application of the clinical judgment model in nursing. *Journal of Nursing Education*, 56(5), 305–308.

Traynor M (2017) *Critical Resilience for Nurses: An Evidence-Based Guide to Survival and Change in the Modern NHS*. London: Routledge.

Tyler T R, Kramer R M and John O P eds (2014) *The Psychology of the Social Self*. Hove: Psychology Press.

Wadsworth P, Colorafi K and Shearer N (2017) Using Narratives to Enhance Nursing Practice and Leadership: What Makes a Good Nurse? *Teaching and Learning in Nursing*, 12(1), 28–31.

Willis P (1979) Shop floor culture, masculinity and the wage form. In Clarke J, Critcher, C and Johnson R (eds) *Working Class Culture: Studies in History and Theory*. London: Hutchinson, 185–198.

Wolf, Z R (2008). Nurses' stories: discovering essential nursing. *MedSurg Nursing*, 17(5), 324.

Wright J (dir) (2007) Atonement. Film. Hollywood: Universal Pictures.

1   Transgressive texts about nursing

Introduction

Popular culture texts can be categorised into the conventional and the transgressive (Fiske, 2010). A conventional text offers a normative view on an issue, a view which is generally acceptable and expected. Many television hospital dramas and soap operas are conventional texts. They typically feature nursing characters who draw heavily from the "good nurse" trope. Such stereotyped portrayals ensure the (female) nurse is placed in the position of assistant to the (male) doctor and that she is caring and selfless. Transgressive texts, on the other hand, violate those norms of the good nurse trope.

As transgressive texts are by nature non-conformist, they can be so subversive as to be shocking. When they are effective, they can challenge restrictive thinking. This is because recognising such representations can lead to better portrayals in the future, and a wider understanding of the complexities of the issue (Ellis, 2014). An example of this is the representations of disabled crime fighters on television. The 1960s series *Ironside* (Young, 1967–1975) featured a detective, played by Raymond Burr in a wheelchair. In television shows like *Law and Order SVU* (Wolf, 1999), when disability prejudice was portrayed and discussed (Zalla, 2008), wide commentary on the issue followed, which in turn inspired more television shows to cover a wider range of disabilities.

Storey (2003) explains that more examples of transgressions about a particular issue in mass culture indicate that a dominant ideology is beginning to waiver in its authority. The notion of being a transgendered individual, for example, transgresses the belief that there are two discrete genders in human biology. Thus, an increasing representation of transgendered characters in popular culture may suggest that the idea of only two genders is, first, under challenge and, then, in the process of being superseded. Transgressions can also be seen as a site of resistance to dominant ideology, where accepted truths are subverted, allowing new thinking on a topic to emerge, possibly eventually prompting change in ideology. Mallett (2009) argues that such moments of transgression are important to identify because, in indicating where conventions have been defied, new ideas and possibilities are also presented for consideration. This can be seen in popular culture, for example in how *The Simpsons*

(Groening, 1989–current) lampoons many accepted truths about contemporary society. In doing so, it calls into question everyday thinking about the nuclear family and the wisdom of authority figures such as teachers, doctors and church officials. It has been remarked that few previous television shows had ever so boldly and iconoclastically made fun of so many sensitive topics (Alberti, 2004). *The Simpsons* provides a vivid demonstration of how transgressive texts can play with conventions and test the status quo. Consumers of transgressive texts often find pleasure in engaging with such narratives.

This pleasure is described by Lacan (1994), as *jouissance* – an intense feeling produced when evading and transgressing the social order – and even, sometimes, gaining pleasure from (others') pain – when the individual is freed, even if only momentarily, from cultural and hierarchical restrictions (Manga, 2003). *Jouissance* is important because it lightens situations that might otherwise be unbearably painful and exposes absurdities of oppressive ideologies (Lacan, 1994; Zizek, 2009). This is why fans and scholars of popular culture find transgressive texts fun, pleasurable and exciting. One such revealing transgressive story, which provides a clear exception to the good nurse trope, is found in the British television series *Getting On* (BBC, 2009–2011).

Getting On

Getting On is set in an English National Health Service (NHS) hospital, in the geriatric ward. The series provides darkly comedic insights into class hierarchies and power inequities between health care workers, and between them and their patients. Written by its core cast, Jo Brand (an ex-nurse turned comedian), Vicki Pepperdine and Joanne Scanlan, the series ran for three seasons in the UK and has been adapted for the American market (HBO, 2013).

The initial episode of the first series opens with an extreme close-up of an old woman's mottled and bandaged hand, setting in place the promise of intimate close-ups of nursing and health care. The hand-held camera glides up to the patient's anguished face, and down to her other hand, which viewers see is being held. The camera pans slowly outward revealing that the person holding the old woman's hand is the Ward Sister, Denise Flixter, who is also known as Den. Den holds a smartphone in her other hand. This is capturing her attention and she is giggling. In this moment, and in stark contrast to Nurse Tallis in *Atonement* (discussed in the Introduction), she clearly defiles a sacred moment and transgresses the trope of the good nurse. While, like Nurse Tallis, she is attending to someone in their final hours, using human connection so that the patient does not have to die alone, her demeanour is totally unlike this paragon's. Den's attention is elsewhere and, despite the solemnity of the scene, she cannot suppress her childish delight at what she is reading on her phone. Then, something makes Den look up from her reverie. The viewer is unsure if this is intuition, or whether she can no longer feel the pulse or hear the breathing of her dying patient. This example from the first few seconds of this series illustrates the shocking power of transgressive texts. It clearly lampoons nursing stereotypes and political correctness. This chapter explores such patent transgressions of the good nurse stereotype and, in doing so, considers what these texts reveal about nursing's place within health care, its on-going struggles for identity and value, and anxieties related to health care. It also illuminates some paradoxes inherent in nursing and its representation.

Aware that her indulgence needs to stop, Den's nursing knowledge comes to the fore and she steps into action as Sister Flixter begins the serious business of caring for the deceased. Before, however, she can make much headway, she is interrupted by a nursing assistant, Kim Wilde, whose statement underscores the transgressive nature of *Getting On*.

> "Den, there's a shit on a chair", Kim states in a deadpan voice.
> Den answers, in an exasperated tone, "It's faeces, not shit".
> Kim rallies with, "There's *faeces* on a chair".
> Den, finishing the repositioning of the deceased patient, refocuses and
>   states, "Okay. Right. Where's this shit? Err ... faeces".

Together the nurses assess the "deposit" on the chair and confirm that it is indeed faeces. Kim volunteers to clean it up, but Den overrules her, saying, "No, Kim. No. That constitutes a critical incident. So, I'm going to call CERIUM [the infection control services] and get them to come and clean the chair. Can you fill in the critical incident form?" The faeces remain on the chair all day, cordoned off with hazard tape, as the nursing team awaits the staff whose job it is to clean up "contaminants". This irreverent scene mocks the irrationality and hypocrisy embedded within nursing culture, in the process calling attention to the politically correct language – "deposit", "hazard", "contaminants" – that serves to separate those who make policy from those who have to implement it (Johnson, 2016).

Sitting with the dying and laying out a deceased body are two rituals that are normally taken very seriously in nursing. But in the plotting, action and dialogue of this episode, these rituals are seen as commonplace and tedious, and also on a par with dealing with faeces and other quotidian, but often disgusting, bodily secretions. The show exposes the nature of nursing work as mundane and unglamorous and, in addition, draws attention to ridiculous policies and bureaucratic dictates that make nurses' work overly complicated and, in some cases, ineffective. The show also reveals how, sometimes, the unrelenting expectation for nurses to be compassionate, attentive and selfless is not always met – whether through human failings or the need to deal with competing demands. In this geriatric ward, mortality is a routine fact of life and faeces on a chair attracts more comment and drama than a patient's death. The nursing staff, like the ward and its patients, are marginalised elements of the hospital system, and it is clear that they realise their work has low status. Thus, in the words of the programme's title, the staff of the unit are simply "getting on"; getting on with work, life, ageing, dying and death.

Kim, the general "dogs-body" nursing assistant is overweight, slow and tired, but she is also kindly and empathic. She does not, however, appear able to make any autonomous decision, no matter how trivial. Her supervising colleague, Sister Flixter, manages the ward competently and appears quite skillful, but is also overweight and slow and shows little empathy for anyone, appearing to be more preoccupied with her troubled personal life than work on the ward. In contrast, the lithe, impeccably dressed Dr. Pippa Moore, with her upper-class accent and unfinished sentences, is helplessly reliant on the nursing staff for direction. Despite her obvious incompetence, she exudes a superior air and strives to make her daily work more interesting by pursuing scientific challenges. In this episode, this involves her trying to improve upon the Bristol Stool Chart – a national tool that classifies human faeces. Meanwhile, she neglects to make the more practical decisions the nursing staff are expecting – and need – from her.

Getting On also comments critically on the supposed policy of equality driving the NHS, the ideology that all UK citizens have a right to access health care. As many reports have revealed, however, elderly patients experience substandard care, neglect and even abuse (Gorman, 2017; MacKenzie, 2017), and many struggle to even access basic medical care (Cohen and Brown, 2013). When those elderly are also members of a racial minority, they are further marginalised. This is reflected in another scene from the second episode of *Getting On*. In this scene, Den, Kim and Dr. Moore, together with her medical students, investigate what is distressing an old Asian-looking woman, who is rambling loudly in a language that no one in the care team can understand. Eventually, Kim is able to contact the hospital's translation service but they cannot attend to consult until the next day. Den suggests that if the nurses convey to the translator over the phone what the old woman is saying, then perhaps he can complete the translation. This results in a farcical interaction. The patient speaks. Den mimics this to Kim: "Gooly-gale-genema", and Kim conveys it to the translator on the phone, "Gooly-gale-genema". The patient continues to speak and Den again attempts to mimic this: "Adga-mortichai". Kim again conveys it: "Adga-mortichai", and then tells the nurse in the room, "He says that first one doesn't mean anything". They persist, relaying "Hannibal-ja-chi" and then being told that this did not mean anything either. Ever-industrious, Den suggests, "Well, listen, what about if you bring the phone up, hold it out there, and he can hear and see if he can translate over the phone?". The patient speaks again. Kim asks, "Hello, did you get that?". This time, however, she has an answer and replies, "Oh, you did? Oh, fantastic. Let me get a pen. Blimey, okay, thanks ever so much. Cheers". When Den asks "Well?", Kim advises that the woman is saying, "I want to die, please kill me." Den, without missing a beat, advises, "Put it in her notes". The *jouissance* in this scene derives from the politically incorrect way the nurses act in their attempt to try to help their elderly patient. At one level, this is simply a beautifully paced comedy of errors. But on another level, it is a radically subversive narrative that exposes the difficulties of ageing and the functional attitude that nurses, many of them female in this area of health care, bring to their work. The nurses are not unkind, but they do not approach their labour as a natural extension of their female identity (Johnson, 2016).

In this scene, *Getting On* poignantly confronts the real and tragic issue of many ageing patients in over-stretched public hospitals. These patients are doubly marginalised; they are frail-aged as well as isolated because of language and ethnicity. At the end of the excruciatingly awkward relay of words, viewers expect to finally understand the ramblings of a confused old lady. What they hear instead is truly shocking. The patient is suicidal and begs the nurses to engage in an act of mercy killing. But rather than acknowledge her extreme emotional state, Den's way of dealing with this drama is to swiftly defuse it with officious action. "Put it in her notes". Again, a functional attitude to nursing is revealed as the nurses proceed to "get on" with their work. Johnson (2016, p. 192) explains that the significance of scenes such as this in the series are to provide an insider's perspective of the "messy, ugly, yet crucial work" completed by the carers in aged care. This and many other scenes throughout the series raise the suggestion that contemporary nurses do not always act, or speak, in ways that conform to the stereotype of "the good nurse". That is, nurses today are not always composed, deferent or compliant. Sometimes they are disengaged, flippant and self-preserving.

Other scenes in *Getting On* allude to unproductive game-playing, class divisions and professional hierarchies, as well as tension between the nurses themselves. In one such scene, the nurses learn that a new "modern matron", Hilary Loftus, has commenced work in the hospital. When he arrives, Den and Kim are taken aback to find that the matron is a man. Overweight, tightly coiled and sexually ambiguous, Hilary does not appear congenial or likely to mix well with the other nurses and he is immediately embroiled in struggles in the ward. He sees an empty bed and claims it for a patient, only to learn that Dr. Moore has already requested it. This pits nurse against doctor. Then, Hilary notices that Den is not wearing regulation footwear, instead sporting ankle boots that he says makes him think of strip clubs. This pits nurse against nurse. Finally, Hilary spies the faeces on the chair and can barely contain his anger, ordering Kim to clean it up immediately. At the bottom of this hierarchy, Kim is caught in a dilemma, knowing she will earn the wrath of Dr. Moore, as well as everyone in the nursing pecking order, whatever action she chooses. Both Kim and Den, the working nurses in the ward, are summarily punished and put in their place, and the matron concludes his visit with one final insult. He suggests that this ward, that the nurses work so solidly to keep in order, has "MRSA [an antibiotic-resistant bacteria] written all over it"!

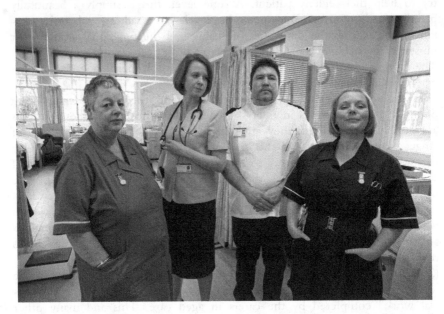

Figure 1.1 The *Getting On* team – barely tolerating each other and the demands of their work.

This transgressive scene playfully makes the gender, class and labour divisions in nursing visible. Men in nursing remain in the vast minority, yet they are over-represented in middle management positions (Limi-nana-Gras et al., 2013). The working-class women, Den and Kim, are viewed scathingly from the moral high ground of the matron who out-ranks them. In a reworking of the "battleaxe stereotype" (Darbyshire and Gordon, 2005; Gillespie et al., 1989), this matron is not buxom but is still oversized, not boisterous but is uptight and quick to make judge-ments about the competence of the nurses, rather than providing any real assistance in terms of the work to be done. This brief scene also comments critically on public health policy. The "modern matron" was a new role and description coined in 2001 in the UK, when the NHS responded to complaints about falling standards in patient care, and par-ticularly in infection control (Shuttleworth, 2004). The role was specific-ally established to give clinical staff much-needed support to achieve improvements. In line with what is portrayed in this scene in *Getting On*, however, the policy added another layer to an already overloaded bureaucracy and has not been particularly successful (Buchanan et al., 2013).

The scene also references the widely known nursing issue of a dominating, bullying culture that leads to lateral, or horizontal, violence (Blair, 2013).

It exposes the sources of irresolvable anxieties for nurses – the constant demand for care from ill and dependent patients, the unexpected intrusions on already overloaded schedules and ever-pressing deadlines, the officious colleagues, and the undercurrents of desire, envy and/or dislike among colleagues. It comments critically on bureaucratic procedures and policies that interfere with nursing work, rather than improve it. In addition, it reveals taboo issues occurring in hospitals every day, but which go unnoticed by everyone except the workers who have inside knowledge: that often patients suffer, that they can struggle to communicate and have their needs met, and that nursing (and medical) work can be simultaneously mundane and disgusting as well as dramatic and awe inspiring.

In this way, this seemingly light comedy provides a rare counter story to the more commonplace and pervasive image of the good nurse. As a transgressive text, *Getting On* shows that nursing is not a romantic occupation or a continually cognitively stimulating profession. Nor is nursing shown to be comprised of altruistic acts of caring leading to self-affirming satisfaction. Instead, *Getting On* presents nursing as hard physical work, much of which is unrecognised and underappreciated. It is also shown to be a profession with very little likelihood of promotion, and where nurses not only have limited resources with which to deal with adverse circumstances, they also have to cope with a disinterested, but intrusive, bureaucracy that is mismanaged at every level. Instead of glamorising and idealising nursing work and nurses, *Getting On* points out the tedious and mundane nature of some nursing labour, and the sometimes-flawed nature of the staff who perform it. Through this lens, viewers may recognise, and come to appreciate, the constraints and inequities that nurses need to endure – excessive bureaucracy, unjust professional hierarchies, marginalisation, difficult personalities and unrelenting hard physical work. All is not completely black, though. *Getting On* also provides glimpses of empathy, compassion, kindness, humour and altruism which effectively humanise both the nurses who perform the work and the profession they belong to.

Nurse Jackie

Another television series, *Nurse Jackie* (Brixius, Dunsky and Wallem, 2009–2015), also provides critical commentary on nurses and nursing through the genre of black comedy. Set in the emergency department of All Saints Hospital in New York City, a fictitious urban Catholic hospital, the 2009 pilot episode was viewed by over one million American viewers (Bednarek, 2015) and, in 2010, Edie Falco won the first of several Emmy Awards for her eponymous leading role. Clearly, the show was engaging for many people and, as such, has the potential to significantly challenge stereotypes about working women more generally and nurses in particular. Like *Getting On*, *Nurse Jackie* does not romanticise nursing, but the series does retain some features of the good nurse trope, in that its protagonist, Nurse Jackie Peyton, is feminine and sexy and most of the nurses in the series are compliant hand-maidens to the doctors. Jackie certainly puts her patients first and demon-strates high standards of care, yet she is also ethically compromised.

In the pilot episode, in agony with back pain, Jackie snorts the powder from drug capsules to get through her shift. She also steals from one patient to give to another, flushes a human ear down the toilet as retribution for that patient's domestic violence and forges a deceased patient's signature in order that he is listed as an organ donor. Each action reveals her individual moral code, which is very different to that of the compliant, rule-following "good nurse". She is also annoyed to learn she has been allocated a student nurse to supervise. The admiring student, Zoey, is unaware of Jackie's addiction, and after working alongside her for a couple of hours, declares Jackie to be a "saint". Jackie later ponders this judgement in a voice-over, stating:

> If I were a saint, which maybe I wanna be, maybe I don't, I would be like Augustine. He knew there was good in him and he knew there was some not so good. And he wasn't going to give up his earthly pleasures before he was good and ready. Make me good, God, but not yet.
>
> (pilot episode, 2009)

This is a subtle parody of St. Augustine's well known prayer, even more meaningful in the context of this series as Augustine is also the patron saint of brewers (Gonzalez, 1987). Not simply "good" nor "bad", saint nor sinner, Nurse Jackie is presented as a complex (that is, human) character. Having become addicted to pain medications so that she can keep working after a workplace injury, her life is disintegrating as her need for the pain killing drug is starting to take precedence over other parts of her life.

Paradoxically, although she works in a values-based hospital, where she could have immediate access to health care, she is reluctant to seek treatment for herself. As the main breadwinner in her working-class family, it is made clear that she could afford neither the time off work nor the cost of the surgery. Under financial pressure, wracked with pain and in denial about her addiction, Jackie also swears often, and is rude to anyone she deems annoying or incompetent. Having an affair with the hospital pharmacist in order to gain access to the prescription pain killers, she also regularly puts her nursing work before her roles as mother and home maker. Yet, she has loyal friends, and the hospital staff and patients deeply respect her high-level skills. She can be compassionate, clinically accurate and decisive in emergencies, and thus – despite her flaws – has the potential to be the epitome of what could be termed a "good nurse" in the contemporary world.

Part of the reason Jackie is so compelling as a character is that, despite this potential, her repeated transgressions of the good nurse trope sets up many opportunities for both dramatic tension and the development of her complex characterisation. Sometimes she acts appallingly to gratify her drug depend-ence and to cover up her lies and deceptions but, in other circumstances, she acts heroically. Where *Getting On* is a social commentary on the systemic failures in health care, *Nurse Jackie* explores a flawed individual whose behaviour is variously outrageous *and* compassionate. In the first episode of Series 3 (2011), for example, an introspective and fearful little boy is brought to the emergency room with some kind of instrument forced up his nose. The team learn that he put it there, trying to see his brain. Dr. Cooper, the assessing doctor who is known to have little empathy or emotional intelligence, cannot remove the foreign object and requests an x-ray. Nurse Jackie, empathising with the little boy's fear and recognising curiosity, persuades Cooper to order a CT scan instead, so that he can be shown a visual picture of his brain. Later, she is seen captivating the boy with a fairytale about the parts of his brain that are responsible for his wisdom and special skills.

Another scene in this episode draws attention to an austere funding climate that is seeing local hospitals closed and nurses rendered unemployed. The nursing director, Gloria Akalitus (appearing in the role of battleaxe matron), convenes an ad hoc meeting around the nurses' station to deliver the news that staff are to expect increased patient demand over the coming weeks. At the same time, she threateningly warns the nurses that the funding situation has produced a glut of nurses on the job market. This means, she advises the nursing staff, who are already exhausted from the seemingly never-ending influx of patients, that they need to lift their game as they are all easily replaced. Unsurprisingly, this does little for morale, however, Jackie, who it is likely has seen such policies come and go in her many years of experience, pays the director no heed and excuses herself to return to the pressing problem at hand – the very ill patients in the emergency department. In this moment, despite her cynicism, Nurse Jackie displays considerable agency. She knows she is a valuable resource and, armed with this sense of her own worth, is able to ignore and transcend the irrational politics and bullying management. Instead, flawed though she may be, she makes a superior moral decision to return to her care role.

Kristy Chambers' memoir

A first-person memoir by Australian nurse Kristy Chambers, *Get Well Soon! My (Un)Brilliant Career as a Nurse* (2012), reveals a dimension of nursing identity that *Nurse Jackie* touches upon but does not elaborate – one that is funny and irreverent. This is used to market the book. In the blurb on the book cover, and in stark contrast to a plethora of memoirs by, or about, stereotypically "good" nurses, Chambers describes her lack of a "calling" and undermines any idea of the nurse as saint or angel:

> My quest for a career started early, when I was four years old and gave myself a haircut to see if I liked that sort of thing. I liked it plenty, but my mother did not. Much later in life, after moonlighting as a maid and enduring myriad other unsatisfying positions, I fell into nursing, the way one may fall into a pile of sheep shit at two in the morning (which I have also done).

This description of her interests and activities prior to nursing lampoons the idea that nurses universally share a background as children with gentle, nurturing temperaments, who then pursue a clearly designated path that leads to nursing (Eley et al., 2012). For Chambers, becoming a nurse was an unhappy accident. Further, her witty similes suggest that Chambers is no demure, shrinking violet and that her memoir is not likely to be a series of nostalgic reflections. It is, rather, a series of anecdotes and stories of disruption and chaos. As such, she describes on the back cover how she felt dazed after her training, an education that had not promoted in her any overwhelming sense of dedication to care:

> Aged thirty, I was spat out of university with a degree in nursing and a sense of bewilderment. I was dumb with wonder: I wondered why on earth I hadn't studied something else, like furniture design. I like chairs.

Chambers then describes the difficulty of her early days in nursing, and – like Nurse Jackie – her own propensity to swear, but then reflects on the inner strength and personal satisfaction she gained from this period in her career:

> My baptism of fire in nursing was harsh, but a pointed reminder that buried beneath my foul mouth was a kind heart, and I had been given an opportunity to use it on a daily basis. I like chairs and sick people. Nursing has been both a hellride and a joyride, but brutally educational most of all.

Chambers thus reveals to even the most casual browser that she had no burning desire to become a nurse, nor any drive to join the profession in order to find work that provided her with an outlet for inherent caring values. Despite this, she acknowledges that nursing has been important to her developing identity – it was, after all, at least in part a "joyride". These brief passages reveal that, like the fictional Nurse Jackie, it is also possible for real nurses to be complex characters; uncouth as well as caring, funny as well as serious, stony as well as sensitive and capable of handling emotional extremes – in other words, complicated and human. Moreover, Chambers' narrative reveals that nursing involves negative – it is, after all, a "hellride" – as well as positive experiences.

In the memoir, Chambers also writes candidly of her own struggle with depression and how this helps her empathise with patients who have mental illness. Despite, or perhaps armed with, this knowledge, she is savvy about how tumultuous working in this area of the health system can be:

> I was diagnosed with depression at 15 and come from a family with a very long, rich history of mental illness. The "crazy" is strong with my people, so I don't use the word with any kind of malice or unkind intention. There is just no other word to cheerfully describe the chaotic atmosphere of an acute mental health ward. "Batshitfuckingcrazytown" would be more apt, at times, but sounds much less friendly.

(p. 17)

In this passage, Chambers reveals something about nursing that is generally hidden from the public and unvoiced in public discourse – that nurses may come from traumatic backgrounds, such as families riven with mental illness – and that, even as they care for others, nurses themselves can be wounded and suffering (Conti-O'Hare, 2002; Heinrich, 1992). Chambers also reveals a largely hidden aspect of hospitals, one that only emerges when system breakdowns are revealed; that, behind the thinly disguised professional veneer presented to the public view, chaos and unreason sometimes reign.

Chambers' narrative also challenges the stereotype that nurses have a bottomless well of sympathy or empathy to share with patients or are constantly engaged with the work at hand. Describing her early days as a nurse, she writes:

> Nothing that dramatic happened. I just found myself cornered all day long by chatty Cathys who had the incredible ability to tell stories that went on and on and on, and at the same time went absolutely nowhere. They would follow me around the ward like sheepdogs, separating me from my preceptor and the rest of the nurse herd so they could get some one-on-one attention and bore my brains out. The days felt extremely long and the only part I really looked forward to was lunch.
>
> (2013, pp. 17–18)

In this manner, Chambers constructs a narratorial nursing self who is empathic but also ironic. Her critical eye reveals much about the hard emotional labour of nursing that is usually hidden from the public, and certainly absent in the image of the "good nurse".

The concept of emotional labour is important to consider in terms of nursing work. Sociologist Hochschild (1983) first defined the term emotional labour as a result of her research on the work of flight attendants, referring to service workers having to regulate their emotions during interactions with clients, fellow workers and their bosses. In relation to nurses, emotional labour is performed in interactions with patients as well as with other nurses, managers and those in superior positions. This regulation includes both the display of emotions that are mandated to be desirable, as well as the suppression of those that are undesirable. This is recognised to involve considerable, although often unacknowledged, skill and effort (Bellas, 1999) and is related to burnout (Brotheridge and Grandey, 2002) and leaving the profession (Cheng et al., 2013). Bellas (1999) notes that greater levels of emotional labour are expected from, and delivered by, women. Chambers' narrative often deftly hints at the requirement in nursing, and in other gendered professions where emotional labour is required, for a degree of both surface acting and deep acting. As Ashforth and Humphrey (1993) explain, surface acting involves simulating emotions such as patience, empathy or even nonchalance, which are not actually felt but which may help the patient to feel as though they are in safe hands.

Deep acting is where real feelings such as boredom and even horror or fear are consciously, and actively, suppressed. Chambers' discussions are valuable as, despite its centrality in practice, and importance in pressing issues such as the high levels of nurses leaving the profession, research reveals that emotional labour remains an under-addressed topic in nursing education and the workforce (Gray, 2009).

Chambers also comments upon another largely unrecognised tendency; that nurses tend to dehumanise or neglect the needs of one another. Dehumanisation can be a consequence of the ongoing emotional distancing that occurs in the everyday work of people in emotional labour-oriented fields (Huy, 1999). The memoir vividly describes how nursing students are herded through their studies and clinical placements, often bored, and regularly left to observe patients or hospital procedures without useful guidance or authentic and scaffolded learning assistance or other advice. Although these observations are supported by recent pedagogical research in the field, they are still not widely acknowledged (Kelly and McAllister, 2013; Shahsavari et al., 2013).

In this vein, Chambers also unsettles the idealised image of the usual location in which nursing takes place: the hospital. Rather than present it as a state-of-the-art scientific site, action-packed with clever, highly trained people rushing to save lives at every turn, she describes the hospital as dreary and bureaucratic – a place where time drags, not unlike how the geriatric ward is represented in *Getting On*. Chambers' is neither a romantic nor an exciting entrée into working life.

> The first week at the hospital was one of the dullest of my life, a long and tedious orientation with mandatory content on occupational health and safety issues and hospital protocol. The speakers were euthanising, the sandwiches were soggy and the coffee was International Roast, which tasted like arse.
>
> (2013, pp. 45–46)

Instead, nursing is dull, long, tedious and unappetising – the poor catering a metaphor for the lack of interest engendered in Chambers during her orientation.

In this passage, Chambers also mocks an enduring signifier for virtuous nursing – the nursing uniform.

> To add insult to injury, I was given my new uniform. It consisted of a fugly blue-and-white floral dress that people called the "libra fleur" because it looked like the outside of a tampon box, a shirt in the same foul material, and navy slacks for cooler weather.
>
> (2013, pp. 45–46)

Once a symbol that connoted precision, hygiene, regulation, order and pro-fessionalism, the white nurses' uniform is, in the contemporary profession, neither practical nor attractive. Decades ago in nursing, donning the pristine uniform was an important *rite de passage* that, like the novitiate becoming a nun, heralded a student's separation from the personal and private (Poovey, 1989), and reminded them that they were about to become "in the world, but not a part of it" (Reverby, 1996). However, since the 1970s, the uniform has been subject to criticism and revision. A white dress not only made the uniform impractical, it also excluded men from the role. Uniform features such as epaulettes, veils, caps and capes were too closely linked to the military and religion and did not suggest a corporate image, a new ideal in keeping with the business ethos sweeping health systems globally in the second half of the twentieth century (Hallam, 2000; Pusey, 1991). Yet, the replacement of the white uniform has not brought with it nursing's emancipation. In her derisive allusion to a tampon box, Chambers suggests that the uniform, and by association the profession it represents, still remains highly gendered, only now, instead of suggesting power and competence, the uniform risks making nurses the brunt of jokes and, moreover, jokes with a lewd edge. In this way, Chambers contests the subject positioning of nursing as corporatised. Readers who share the joke with her may empathise with a nursing struggle that seeks a professional identity carved more from the work entailed and its requisite skills and knowledge, than by its more exterior and frivolous aspects. The nursing identity performed in this transgressive text is also well aware of the task involved, as well as the cost, of the emotional labour expected and executed in the course of nursing.

Transgressive representations of nursing

The texts considered in this chapter are unusual in that they foreground nurses' experiences in ways that are clearly critical of the current dominant ideology in health care. Den and Kim get the job done in their ward despite the hospital's policies and the self-important Dr. Moore. Nurse Jackie may not have everything in her life "together", but she does have compassion for patients, and her nursing is empathic and patient-centred. Kristy Chambers was under no illusion that her inherent qualities (as a woman, and gained from the sum of her past human experience) made her a better nurse. These narratives also reveal the sheer hard work involved in nursing. Each text shows that while nursing is complex and demanding cognitive work, requir-ing multiple clinical decisions to be made every minute, there are also repeti-tive tasks that are boring and taxing and, as a result, exhausting. The expectation that nurses repress their own feelings in order to put their patients' needs first is also clearly portrayed.

Each of these transgressive texts also portrays how everyday nursing work involves hidden struggles that are often unnoticed – and unremarked – by others. The representation of nurses in these works reveals the nursing profession to be a divided and oppressed group that is overly hierarchical and managerial. Nurses are frequently ignored by doctors who see themselves as superior, and it is hard for nurses to have their say and also be respected. These texts also challenge the idea that nursing is women's work, revealing that nursing is hard work, but the nature of that work is not domestic or feminine. Although women continue to dominate the profession in terms of numbers, they are marginalised and oppressed because of their gender.

It is paradoxical that these departures from the entrenched idea of the "good" nurse are examined so deeply and provocatively in popular culture, yet are rarely mentioned or discussed in either the professional nursing literature or nursing education. Further, despite being able to be categorised as light entertainment, the subject matter with which these texts deal is weighty. This has not escaped commentary outside the world of nursing. *Getting On* has been described as a "radical, profound masterpiece" (Orr, 2012) for how it portrays the world of work, and *Nurse Jackie* has been nominated for many television awards and continues to be watched and discussed (Bednarek, 2015). Chambers' memoir was published by a leading Australian university press and has been of interest to feminist scholars (McAllister and Brien, 2015).

Conclusion

This chapter has focused on popular culture texts that transgress commonplace, taken for granted understanding of nurses. It is transgressive to suggest that nurses may have limits to their caring capacities or may make mistakes. Transgressive texts about nursing also reveal that there is not simply one universal way, or narrative, to describe or explain, nursing in society. Transgressive texts suggest, instead, that nurses and nursing are complex and multi-layered, and worthy of deeper consideration.

Getting On, *Nurse Jackie* and *Get Well Soon* are thus significant because they provide a counter-narrative to simplistic and idealised beliefs that nurses are always demure, caring and devoted to their vocation. Each of these works provides a clear critique of contemporary nursing and the way gender, class, ageing and health care hierarchies affect how nursing is performed. Despite their humorous tone, these narratives reveal deep truths about the emotional labour expected, and performed, by nurses and the cost nurses pay in this performance. They also expose neo-liberal managerialism as a discourse that separates health care policy makers from frontline workers and hinders the safe and empathic care of patients. These entertaining texts, therefore, reveal a profound awareness and appreciation of complexity and imperfection. For those with a knowledge of nursing history, these narratives powerfully illustrate that nursing is a social construct that is shaped and constrained by changing social needs and attitudes. The issues that were imperative in the days of Florence Nightingale – to use standard ways of working, and to use nursing as a means to elevate the status of (at least some) women – have developed in complexity.

Revealing such transgressions through popular cultural representation is also potentially consciousness raising and may lead to change. This is because, when nurses and others become aware of how such norms and conventions are being played with, and subverted, they may also become more informed about what really occurs in nursing. Such stories provide important counter-points to powerful, dominant ideologies by revealing tensions and contradictions in the prevailing assumptions that underpin those ideologies. The next chapter in this book explores a series of narratives that uncover additional complexities and paradoxes about nursing.

References

Alberti J (ed) (2004) *Leaving Springfield: The Simpsons and the Possibility of Oppositional Culture*. Detroit: Wayne State University Press.

Ashforth B and Humphrey R (1993) Emotional labour in service roles: The influence of identity *Academy of Management Review* 18(1): 88–115.

Bednarek M (2015) "Wicked" women in contemporary pop culture: "Bad" language and gender in *Weeds, Nurse Jackie*, and *Saving Grace Text & Talk* 35(4): 431–451.

Bellas M (1999) Emotional labour in academia: The case of professors *ANNALS of the American Academy of Political and Social Science* 561: 96–110.

Blair P (2013) Lateral violence in nursing *Journal of Emergency Nursing* 39(5): e75–e78.

Brand J, Pepperdine V and Scanlan J (2009–2012) *Getting On*. Television series. London: BBC.

Brixius L, Dunsky E and Wallem L (creators) (2009–2015) *Nurse Jackie*. Television series. Hollywood: Showtime.

Brotheridge C and Grandey A (2002) Emotional labor and burnout: Comparing two perspectives of people work *Journal of Vocational Behavior* 60: 17–39.

Buchanan D, Parry E, Gascoigne C and Moore C (2013) Are healthcare middle management jobs extreme jobs? *Journal of Health Organization and Management* 27(5): 646–664.

Chambers K (2013) *Get Well Soon: My Unbrilliant Career as a Nurse*. St Lucia: University of Queensland Press.

Cheng C, Bartram T, Karimi L and Leggat S (2013) The role of team climate in the management of emotional labour: Implications for nurse retention *Journal of Advanced Nursing* 69(12): 2812–2825.

Cohen T and Brown L (2013) Care home covered up neglected that killed five: Staff shredded medical records revealing 'institutional abuse'. *Daily Mail*, 18 October. Available at: www.dailymail.co.uk/news/article-2465955/Five-elderly-residents-died-neglect-care-home-institutionalised-abuse.html.

Conti-O'Hare M (2002) *The Nurse as Wounded Healer: From Trauma to Transcendence*. New York: Jones and Bartlett.

Darbyshire P and Gordon S (2005) Exploring popular images and representations of nurses and nursing. In Daly J, Speedy S D, Jackson D, Lambert V and Lambert C (eds) *Professional Nursing: Concepts, Issues and Challenges*. New York: Springer, 69–92.

Eley D, Eley R, Bertello M and Rogers-Clark C (2012) Why did I become a nurse?: Personality traits and reasons for entering nursing *Journal of Advanced Nursing* 68(7): 1546–1555.

Ellis K (2014) Cripples, bastards and broken things: Disability in *Game of Thrones M/C Journal* 17(5). Available at: www.journal.media-culture.org.au/index.php/mcjournal/article/view/895.

Fiske J (2010) *Understanding Popular Culture*. London: Routledge.

Gillespie R, McInnes L, Priest D and Langbein I (1989) *Handmaidens and Battleaxes*. Film. Sydney: Silver Films.

Gonzalez J (1987) *A History of Christian Thought: From the Protestant Reformation to the Twentieth Century*, Vol. 3. Nashville: Abingdon Press.

Gorman M (2017) Development and the rights of older people. In Randel J, German T and Ewing D (eds) *The Ageing and Development Report: Poverty, Independence and the World's Older People*. London: Routledge, 69–92.

Gray B (2009) The emotional labour of nursing: Defining and managing emotions in nursing work *Nurse Education Today* 29(2): 168–175.

Groening M (creator) (1989–current) *The Simpsons*. Animated television series. Los Angeles: Fox Broadcasting Company.

Hallam J (2000) *Nursing the Image: Media, Culture and Professional Identity*. London: Routledge.

Heinrich K (1992) Create a tradition: Teach nurses to share stories *Journal of Nursing Education* 31(3): 41–143.

Hochschild A (1983) *The Managed Heart*. Berkeley: University of California Press.

Huy Q (1999) Emotional capability and corporate change *Mastering Strategy* 6: 32–34.

Johnson B (2016) *Getting On*: Ageing, mess and the NHS *Critical Studies in Television* 11(2): 190–203.

Kelly J and McAllister M (2013) Lessons students and new graduates could teach: How to build a supportive learning culture in health services *Contemporary Nurse* 44(2): 170–177.

Lacan J (1994) *The Four Fundamental Concepts of Psycho-Analysis*. Philadelphia: W W Norton.

Liminana-Gras R, Sánchez-López M, Román A and Corbalán-Berná F (2013) Health and gender in female-dominated occupations: The case of male nurses *The Journal of Men's Studies* 21(2): 135–148.

McAllister M and Brien D L (2015) Narratives of the "not-so-good nurse": Rewriting nursing's virtue script *Hecate* 41(2&3): 79–97.

MacKenzie J (2017) ALRC elder abuse inquiry: Recommendations for reform of aged care laws *Bulletin (Law Society of South Australia)* 39(7): 36–37.

Mallett R (2009) Choosing "stereotypes": Debating the efficacy of (British) disability-criticism *Journal of Research in Special Educational Needs* 9(1): 4–11.

Manga J (2003) *The Cultural Politics of Daytime TV Talk Shows*. New York: New York University Press.

Olsen M and Scheffer W (2013) *Getting On*. New York: HBO.

Orr D (2012) *Getting On* isn't just funny: It's radical, profound, a masterpiece. *The Guardian* 23 November. Available at: www.theguardian.com/commentisfree/2012/nov/23/getting-on-bbc4-funny-radical-profound.

Poovey M (1989) *Uneven Developments: The Ideological Work of Gender in Mid-Victorian England*. London: Virago.

Pusey M (1991) *Economic Rationalism in Canberra: A Nation-Building State Changes Its Mind*. Sydney: Cambridge University Press.

Reverby S (1996) *Ordered To Care: The Dilemma Of American Nursing, 1850–1945*. Cambridge: Cambridge University Press.

Shahsavari H, Yekta Z, Houser M and Ghiyasvandian S (2013) Perceived clinical constraints in the nurse student-instructor interactions: A qualitative study *Nurse Education in Practice* 13(6): 546–552.

Shuttleworth A (2004) The role of modern matrons in raising standards of infection control *Nursing Times* 100(26): 61–63.

Storey J (2003) *Inventing Popular Culture: From Folklore to Globalization.* Malden: Blackwell.

Wolf D (creator) (1999) *Law and Order: Special Victims Unit.* Television series. New York: NBC.

Young C (creator) (1967–1975) *Ironside.* Television series. New York: NBC.

Zalla C (dir) (2008) (Inconceivable). *Law & Order: Special Victims Unit.* Television series. New York: NBC.

Zizek S (2009) *First as Tragedy, Then as Farce.* London: Verso.

2 Nursing's dark past and secret knowledge

Introduction

As an almost universally recognised (Donelan et al., 2008) and trusted (Ozaras and Abaan, 2016) profession, nurses have long been admired for the care-giving work that they perform that benefits so many people. This caring role is, indeed, at the heart of the "good nurse" trope which is so entrenched. But a dark part of nursing's and midwifery's history, that spanned the fourteenth to the seventeenth centuries across Europe and North America, is their association with witchcraft. As Ehenreich and English (2010, p. 19) say in their landmark text on this topic:

> The witch hunts left a lasting effect . . . an aura of contamination has remained especially around the midwife and other women healers. This early and devastating exclusion of women from independent healing roles was a violent precedent and a warning: It was to become a theme of our history.

Nurses – mostly women, but about one-fifth of whom were men – could be accused of witchcraft if they had "magical healing powers" (Briggs, 1996). They were often charged specifically with possessing medical and obstetrical skills – something that was the exclusive realm of medical men. Prior to the Enlightenment, healers – including surgeons and physicians – had no medical scientific knowledge to draw upon. At the time, medical students were scholarly young gentlemen who studied Plato, Aristotle and Christian theology and who spent very little time with patients, because the body was considered dirty and soiled and thus any association with it was degrading. Nurses and midwives, on the other hand, visited the sick regularly and tried numerous treatments, in the process gaining vast experience of these conditions and their management. Their knowledge was drawn from a range of arenas: experience, commonsense, herbalism and folk-wisdom passed down from old women to their apprentices. The witch hunts, however, led to widespread betrayal and suppression. It is estimated that 100,000 women were tortured and executed throughout this atrocity and many more lost their only source of income. The example of Jacoba Felicie (also known as Jacqueline Felice de Almania) is illustrative. Brought to trial in 1322 in Paris, she was charged with the following:

she would cure her patient of internal illness and wounds or of external abscesses. She would visit the sick assiduously and continue to examine the urine in the manner of physicians, feel the pulse, and touch the body and limbs.

(Ehenreich and English, 2010, p. 54)

Her crime, it would seem, was to be doing what only male doctors were permitted to do. Although not burned at the stake, she was threatened with excommunication, fined a hefty sum and prohibited from practicing her healing art (Green, 2006).

Throughout these long centuries, anything doctors failed to cure, but nurses and midwives could ameliorate, was derided as sorcery. At this time, male physicians were understood to preside over moral and intellectual domains while the female healer was placed on the side of darkness, evil and magic. Even so, villagers needed these healers and sought them out regularly. Herein lies a paradox that is persistent today – on the one hand, nurses and midwives can be derided or looked upon suspiciously for their knowledge, and use, of what could be called folk-wisdom, yet they also enjoy the trust, respect and sometimes awed regard of patients (Donahue, 1985) for implementing that same knowledge.

An example of this kind of knowledge implementation can be seen in a nurse's response to a dying patient who asked her if her family would remember her when she was gone. The nurse responded not with a platitude, but with another question, designed to ignite thought, imagination and expression (Carlile, 2013). She asked her patient how she would like them to remember her. This question led to the patient creating a portfolio of recordings ranging from family stories to personal letters and words of wisdom the patient wanted to share with family members. This nurse knew, from her education, training and experience on the wards, about the importance of distress prevention during palliative care. She also knew about the stages of dying. What such scientific data could not tell her was the "right" answer to this patient's direct question. Thus, instead of scientific objective reasoning, she used intuition, curiosity and empathic personal engagement to try to understand what problem underlay that question, and provide a solution for the patient. Such interchanges often may, moreover, occur at the same time as scientifically based treatments (such as medicines, injections or dressing changes) are being delivered by nurses.

In addition to this subjective/objective dialectic in nursing knowledge, hierarchical differences in the knowledge domains between nursing and medicine persist, and this cements status differences. After struggling for legitimacy in the eighteenth and nineteenth centuries, both professions now enjoy a high regard within society in terms of being trusted and respected, but nursing in the main remains a solidly working-class occupation, while doctors and surgeons are part of society's elite. Despite both professions requiring tertiary-level training, doctors are widely thought of as highly educated and skilled "thinkers", while nurses are considered practical "doers" (Wicks, 1998). In reality, both doctors and nurses must think and do and, for each of these health care professions, the lines between thought and action (and between science and art), are blurred. Many nurses, for example, hold research higher degrees in nursing and continue to be researchers as well as practitioners (Petty, Cross and Stew, 2012). Similarly, many doctors value and pursue the development of the use of the arts in their profession – the approach known as narrative medicine (Charon, 2008; Mullangi, 2013). Having developed a sense of humility in terms of the limits of their technical skills, such doctors know that despite all the benefits that science can make to a patient's status, that person's unique and human response to suffering, sorrow, beauty and grace are likely to be the major determinants of how well they adapt to their health crisis (Shafer, 2017). This is clearly apparent in physicians' own illness memoirs, where the value of storytelling is understood as enriching in terms of reflecting upon life as a care-giver and in coming to terms with their illness (see, Kalanithi, 2016; O'Brien, 2008). Despite the high esteem in which nursing is held, those in the nursing profession have not been as successful as those in medicine in explaining the scope and intricacies of the art and science of their practice. Although the profession is highly visible in society, public knowledge about nurses and nursing remains shallow (Morris-Thompson et al., 2011).

The analysis in this chapter explores a component of nursing practice which is rarely articulated in research, professional discussion, nursing education or other realms: the mysterious and secret nature of nursing knowledge. It suggests that important aspects of nursing knowledge, those involving intuition, emotion, compassion and kindness, may be inadequately disseminated through textbooks and classroom-teaching, but they are modelled by excellent practitioners and in some powerful storytelling that conveys the essence of what it can mean to effectively nurse a person through an illness, or midwife a woman through to birth. The presentation of nursing knowledge in the television series *Outlander* (Moore, 2014–current) and *Call the Midwife* (Thomas, 2012–current), the classic film *Sister Kenny* (Nichols, 1946) and two personal memoirs, *The Language of Kindness* (Watson, 2018) and *A Nurse's Story* (Shalof, 2005), is explored to discern the complex ways of knowing of a series of very different nurse characters.

Nursing knowledge as mysterious

It is 1947 and Halloween in the Scottish Highlands, where, Celtic legend has it, witches and ghosts are free to roam. The *Samhain* (summer's end) ritual is about to begin. *Samhain* marks the harvest and the approach of dark, cold winter, symbolising the boundary between the world of the living and that of the dead. People build large bonfires and coat their thresholds with chicken blood to protect their homes from evil spirits.

Claire Fraser, a visiting English nurse who has witnessed the ravages of the Second World War, is reminded by the villagers that as a foreigner, an "outlander" as they call her, she will be treated with suspicion. Exploring the atmospheric standing stones at Craigh na Dun, Claire suddenly finds herself hurtled back two centuries to 1743, into the middle of a skirmish between English redcoats and rebel Scottish Highlanders. Soon she realises that not only is she an English outsider in this time, but she is also an outsider in terms of her knowledge, which includes her expertise in health care. The scientific knowledge she has, including of germ theory, infection control, pain relief and wound care, is unknown in this world and seen as suspect and even evil in this much more superstitious era. While her exotic beauty and feisty character distinguish Claire as unusual and alluring, she is also feared because she has access to health care knowledge that is completely foreign to the people of this time. As this knowledge is revealed, the initial suspicions the Highlanders hold about her outsider status deepen, but they are simultaneously drawn to, as well as deterred by, her skills and expertise.

Claire's suspect status is exposed soon after her arrival, when she intervenes to stop a group of rebels from breaking the arm of one of their wounded comrades. While his friends think the bone needs to be fractured to heal, Claire makes a rapid diagnosis – his shoulder is dislocated – and takes swift control to prevent further injury and pain. Ordering the men to back away, she informs the terrified patient of the treatment required and, through the clarity of her explanation and her forceful, confident manner, gains his trust and consent, and then competently forces the dislocated bones back into place. With her patient now relieved of the searing pain, she applies a sling, prescribes warm compresses and then stands back. The other men look on, at first relieved, but remaining suspicious. How can such an insignificant, young and outwardly fragile woman have the knowledge and the skills to contain a situation that was beyond these powerful, experienced men?

Claire embodies some characteristics of the good nurse trope – she is feminine and caring, for instance – but her imaging in the series also suggests that nurses have access to expert (and secret) knowledge that singles them out in society as simultaneously deserving of respect, yet also suspicion. In this way, the representation of the nurse in *Outlander* transgresses the good nurse stereotype and, in doing so, clearly reveals a darker dimension to nursing. This darker dimension is that nurses – by virtue of their medical and surgical experience, as well as their proximity to a space that rests between the sacred and profane – makes them admired, but also enigmatic.

In 1978, Carper proposed four ways to categorise nursing knowledge, and this classification is still utilised today to teach nursing students to be aware that skillful nursing practice requires more than scientific knowledge and correct technique. It also requires an awareness of context, and an elegant delivery of (technical) skills that allays a patient's tension, facilitates trust and builds that patient's confidence (Johns, 1995; Pearson, 2013; White, 1995). Carper's classification includes empirical, ethical, personal and aesthetic ways of knowing. Nurses use empirical knowledge, such as facts and research, to direct actions. In the above scene from *Outlander*, Claire uses her knowledge of anatomy to know what to do to relocate the humerus into the glenoid capsule. Similarly, ethical knowledge is drawn from agreed and evidence-derived principles to ensure that nurses' actions are justified, moral and acceptable. Claire could have remained passive, and watched the man's arm being broken, but she felt a duty to intervene and assist. Claire also drew upon personal knowledge gleaned from her past experiences. She could see that the well-meaning friends were about to attempt something she knew to be incorrect, and would likely cause more injury and extreme pain, trauma and possibly death for the injured man. Undoubtedly, Claire's experience as a war nurse had exposed her to what the ravages of traumatic injury and late treatment could do to a patient.

Importantly, Claire also draws on knowledge in the aesthetic realm, known as the "art" of nursing. Prior to intervening, Claire assessed the context. Faced with the unnerved and adrenaline-charged men, she knew that the manner in which she declared her authority would be all-important. If she could gain their permission, and their capitulation, to work on the patient, she could save his life. If she could gain his trust, he would allow her to perform the manoeuvre necessary to relocate the bone. She commanded that authority in her unwavering eye-contact and determined stance. This embodied what Carper (1978), as well as Nightingale (1860) and many others (Donahue, 1985; Jenner, 1997), have described as the "finest of arts". As Nightingale wrote in 1859: "Health is not only to be well, but to use well every power we have" (p. 186). To achieve this for patients requires creativity and skill, and this therapeutic approach holds true today. As demonstrated so well by Claire, it demands intelligent responsiveness, a willingness to move towards suffering (rather than away from it) and a timely use of skills. Nursing is a fine art because the skilled actions involved blend sensitivity, courage, imagination, empathy, the repression of one's own fears or needs and precise movement/s (Hegge, 2011). When (with her 1947 knowledge) Claire suggests that the patient might feel more comfortable if hot compresses are applied to the damaged area in the days ahead, her knowledge draws upon what could be characterised as a "feeling state" – that is, a combination of empathy, personal knowledge and intuition – rather than strong evidence. It is in this realm where suspicion of nursing knowledge arises.

Numerous scholars argue that aesthetics is what establishes nursing's uniqueness within the health landscape (Edwards, 1998; Eriksson, 2002; Wainright, 2000). Dictionary definitions of aesthetics relate to ideas of beauty and its appreciation, and often in the context of the fine arts (such as music, painting and so forth), but the philosopher Gadamer (2004) provides a fuller descriptive account that relates to the observation and insight that underpins that appreciation. In Gadamer's depiction, aesthetics is a form of perception that harnesses "pure seeing and pure hearing" to produce meaning (p. 92). In this sense, aesthetics is a valuing of subjective knowledge. What the individual as observer sees, and listener hears, regardless of what others may be sensing, is – in this paradigm – legitimate, and can be trusted and interpreted as a knowledge source in order to come to conclusions, and to make meaning about the world. The ancient Greeks applied this aesthetic knowledge to the art of healing, understanding it as the ability to re-establish balance in health and wellbeing for the afflicted (Austgard, 2006). Nightingale had a similar view, writing in 1860 that "nature alone cures ... what nursing has to do ... is to put the patient in the best condition for nature to act upon him" (as cited in Dossey et al., 2005, p. 143). Here Nightingale is suggesting that one of the roles of nursing is that of gently reorienting the patient so that healing can take place, and facilitating balance so that body, mind and spirit can be restored.

Much more than just the prescription of a scientifically determined medical treatment, what can be described as aesthetic practice involves anticipating, and weighing up, the probable outcomes for the patient, and what more – or less – might be needed to achieve balance. Gadamer (2004) explains that when such knowledge is applied to health care, it refers not to the technical procedures performed by the nurse, but to the effect that is produced by nursing, in terms of patient comfort, satisfaction and self-knowledge. This means that aesthetic knowledge includes consideration of the patient's actual condition (not just what is generally predicted from the diagnosis) and their individual experience of illness (rather than the general experience). In the scene from *Outlander*, Claire seems to provide no more or, importantly, no less care than what is required for the soldier to be relieved of pain and, therefore, able to join his fellow Highlanders as soon as possible. While aesthetic knowledge is important to Claire (and – by extrapolation, this scene subtly makes a case for – perhaps for all nurses of her era), the Scottish rebels look at Claire with incredulity. How does she know these things? How can it be that a woman, an outsider foreigner, with no spells or potions, can be more effective than they?

Such rhetorical questions resonate today when nursing knowledge comes to the fore, in the face of – and sometimes in contrast to – other knowledge that could be classified as more scientific. Apparent in this scene of Claire attending to the dislocated shoulder, as elsewhere throughout *Outlander*, is the idea that some of the knowledge nurses use is not always explicable or obvious to others. Such nursing knowledge combines empathy, intuition, imagination and responding to the emotional reactions of others. When understood in this way, nurses, and the care they provide through nursing, can seem mysterious and unknowable. Mirroring the way that the wounded rebel and his companions reacted to Claire and her successful treatment of the dislocated shoulder, nurses are respected for their perception, judgements and actions (and the results flowing from these), but also feared.

Practising ethical ways of knowing

Call the Midwife (Thomas, 2012–current), a BBC television series based on the three first-person memoirs of a community nurse (Worth, 2002, 2005, 2009), is a British period drama about a group of nurses and midwives who deliver community- and hospital-based care in London's East End during the 1950s and 1960s. The seventh episode of the fifth series (Martin, 2016) is set in the early 1960s when the birth defects caused by Thalidomide – a drug prescribed during pregnancy – were gradually revealing themselves and threatening to erupt in a social and health scandal. Although somewhat successful in counteracting the symptoms of morning sickness, Thalidomide caused limb, heart and eye malformations in the developing foetus, and only fifty percent of babies survived. As the surviving children grew, they faced lifetimes of stigma and struggle due to their obvious physical disabilities (Cuthbert, 2003). The third episode in this series used this ethical controversy as the basis for its narrative.

The nurses and midwives in this episode, some – but not all – of whom are Anglican nuns, struggle with the inhumane way that the malformed babies were treated following delivery, which, essentially, ensured that they died. The following scene reveals the distress they felt.

Three nuns gather in the chapel for quiet reflection. Sister Julienne has recently attended the birth of a child born with no limbs, who was left to die by an open window, and is fretting about what she should say to the child's mother.

SISTER JULIENNE: I saw a baby lost today. It was brutal and unbearable. I'm not sure if I did enough. Sister Monica Joan, do you ever think it is acceptable to tell a lie?

SISTER MONICA JOAN SMILES EMPATHICALLY, HOLDS HER HAND AND SAYS: I think the question is not if it's acceptable but if it is kind.

SISTER JULIENNE: I don't know. But I do know that telling the truth would be cruel.

SISTER MONICA JOAN: Then there can be no virtue in it.

SISTER JULIENNE REPLIES, COMFORTED AND NOW KNOWING WHAT SHE MUST NEXT DO: No.

The situation, and the treatment of the child, offended these nurses' values, ethics and the empathic way of knowing that they held so highly. They knew, instinctively and intuitively, that the situation was complex, but were also uncomfortable with how it had been played out and their roles in it. Even so, they had the courage to remain in the situation and to encounter what would have been horrendous. In the next scene, Sister Julienne approaches the mother to deliver the news.

MOTHER: When can I see my baby?

SISTER JULIENNE: Ruby. I'm so very sorry, but your poor little baby was born so desperately unwell that it wasn't possible for us to save it.

MOTHER: It died?

SISTER JULIENNE: Yes, Ruby. In my arms.

MOTHER, UPSET: Was it a girl?

SISTER JULIENNE: pausing because the sex was unable to be determined: Yes.

MOTHER, STRUGGLING: Did she cry?

SISTER JULIENNE: A little. But when she took her last breath she was warm and safe and I believe she was aware that she was loved.

The mother weeps, expressing her grief, and is supported by the nurse.

These moving excerpts highlight the ways of knowing in nursing practice that preceded the preference for technical-rational knowledge which proliferated in, and since, the biotechnology boom of the 1990s. Technical-rationalism emphasises empirical knowing, and nurses are depicted displaying this knowledge in contemporary dramas such as *The Good Doctor* (2017) and *The Resident* (2018). Such representations are presented with high drama and fast-paced action, which has eclipsed the other aspects of nursing knowledge that are perhaps less visual and slower paced. In contrast, a nurse considering difficult choices in an ethical dilemma or sitting with a patient who grieves a dead child are practices that embody what is understood to be the "art" of nursing. A vivid example is offered in Christie Watson's memoir, where she explains it was not books or academic theories that taught her how to nurse, but a memory from her childhood, when, very ill, a nurse showed her compassion and personal care. She writes:

> I had pneumonia; and subsequent anaphylactic reactions to the antibiotics, and how my only sustaining memory from that time – aged eight, when I can well remember other incidents – is of a nurse who fed me orange yoghurt, very slowly, tiny spoonful after tiny spoonful. I remember nothing of the doctors who healed me, but I can still remember the taste of that orange yoghurt.
>
> (2018, p. 112)

This art can often involve courageously moving into, or staying in, a moment of suffering and thus creating a connection that conveys to a patient that suffering can be borne.

Returning to the *Call the Midwife* episode discussed earlier, another midwife is having an (albeit quite veiled) discussion with the doctor in charge about letting another Thalidomide-affected baby die. She initially defers to the doctor, seeking his advice and his decisions regarding the treatment plan, which involves the baby being institutionalised and, probably, soon dying. Later, however, she is also willing to support the mother in order for her to make the decision to accept, and decide to care for, the baby. Of her own volition, the midwife also takes on the task of going to talk to the father who had, at that stage, rejected the child. This is where her full scope of nursing knowledge comes into play for, although there was nothing she could offer the father in terms of medical treatment, she could identify, both rationally and intuitively, that this was a loving and economically secure family that could care for the baby if they made that decision. She understood that for the child to have any chance of health and a decent life, it needed both the community-based care that the family could offer, plus the funds brought in from the father's job. While the doctor saw only the problem ahead (health and otherwise), the nurse was able to use her combined ways of knowing in order to see the big picture, and use both logic and empathy to see that the father could become an ally in the child's care, if she could make a connection with him at this important moment.

In this, she is empowered to act by her own perception and understanding of the situation. The nurse uses knowledge to assert her agency and, in doing so, she is no longer in a dependent relationship with the doctor. This fortifies her commitment to further assist with the situation. For example, her care for the child and her family inspires the other midwives to alter some clothes for the affected baby, so that these will fit her properly. At this time, the midwife mentions that these were clothes thrown away by others and weren't "good enough for little Susan". This is notable too, as the midwife calls the child by its own name, "Susan", rather than referring to it by the more generalised term, "the baby". This moves the child from being a nameless foundling to someone with her own identity. In this, the midwife can be seen to be voicing the move from the institutionalised, uniform care of the past to the more individualised, person-focused care of the future. The basis for such care has to be, in part, based on nurses and other health care professionals being willing to understand the patient as an individual with their own needs, personality and potential, rather than a health condition (McCormack and McCance, 2011). In this episode, and many others in the *Call the Midwife* series and the memoirs they are based on, the nurses and midwives bring more than empirical and technical knowledge to this understanding; they bring their personal experience, empathy and ethical decision-making ability, as well as their aesthetic knowledge that helps to create a context for the expression of suffering and the acceptance of comfort. Using this knowledge wisely takes courage and skill. Actions taken may not be considered compliant or obedient, indeed they may involve defiance and resistance, which may not always be immediately understood or appreciated. As seen in this episode of *Call the Midwife*, nurses may need to transgress accepted order for the highest standards of care to be provided.

Practising critical thinking and having the courage of one's convictions

It is clear, then, that nursing knowledge is not straightforward. Nursing's struggle for legitimacy in terms of this unique way of knowing, and some of the reasons for its suppression, derision and marginalisation is exemplified in a film released not long after the end of the Second World War, *Sister Kenny* (Nichols, 1946). This biopic, based on the life and work of Elizabeth Kenny, provides a romanticised although, paradoxically, mostly accurate account (Ross, 1983) of the Australian nurse who spent over thirty years nursing patients in Toowoomba, Townsville and Brisbane. Kenny nursed in private nursing homes that she set up for the treatment of patients. Most famously, she developed heat and exercise treatments to relieve the symptoms of infantile paralysis, or Poliomyelitis (known today as "Polio") which, at the time, was a highly contagious disease with no known cure. The accepted treatment was immobilisation, which Kenny not only believed to cause pain, muscle wasting and permanent disability, but which was also, in her opinion, avoidable. In a pivotal scene in the film, illustrating the core conflict between her nursing knowledge and established medical procedure, Kenny enters the classroom of a renowned Australian Poliomyelitis specialist physician and commences a heated debate with him exposing their conflicting ideas. Kenny has been warned not to use medical language, such as the word "spasm", which might inflame the ire of the medical professionals, who would see this as a breach of her (nursing) scope of practice.

DR. BRACK: Nurse Kenny, please explain your theory.

SR. KENNY: Well, the fundamental difference between us is which muscle is sick.

DR. BRACK: Go on.

SR. KENNY: Dr. Brack, I didn't expect to find you so tolerant. This is the first time in twenty years I have been given a hearing before orthopaedic men.

DR. BRACK: Yes, Yes, Sister Kenny, go on.

SR. KENNY: Well, Dr. Brack considers that one muscle is paralysed and the opposing muscle is healthy. I say the opposing muscle is sick – in spa … – well, call it a muscle condition. The first thing you must do is to apply moist heat, and to reduce the spa … – the muscle condition. The first thing to do is to keep the muscles relaxed. If you keep them in splints you only make the muscle spasm worse.

DR. BRACK: Yes, that would be quite reasonable if your concept were correct. Come to the convalescent stage …

SR. KENNY: Well, after the spasm …

DR. BRACK INTERRUPTS, APPALLED: Spasm?

SR. KENNY (EXASPERATED): Yes, spasm! After the spasm is relieved, you may find the muscles normal, but they are not. They are alienated, uncoordinated and they need re-education!

DR. BRACK: There is no such thing as spasm in infantile paralysis. Incoordination? Re-education? Alienation? Why, you'll find that word in the divorce court, not in medical science. These are not scientific terms, they are gibberish you invented!

SR. KENNY: Yes, for a new concept, new ideas need new words. The words I use describe the things I see!

DR. BRACK: Well, how is it that we don't see them?

SR. KENNY: Because you've got a book in front of your eyes. Whole libraries, words. If you were interested you wouldn't quibble about the words I use.

DR. BRACK: Without the strict and careful use of words, there would be no science. We can't waste any more time if you express yourself with terms that have no meaning.

SR. KENNY: They have meaning for me. I call it spasm. I treat spasm!

DR. BRACK, MOCKINGLY: And you get cures, isn't that right?

SR. KENNY: Lots of doctors have tried to catch me on that one. I don't claim to have a cure. But I get improvements Doctor, even with your failures.

Written almost seventy years ago, this powerful scene vividly illustrates the clash in cultures between evidence-based medicine and the knowledge gained by both observation and tapping into more experiential, personal knowing about medical treatments and their effects. It reveals how Sister Kenny relies on her sense of sight, smell and "gut" feelings, alongside more objective clinical measures, to detect symptoms and abnormalities. It also expresses how Kenny did possess the scientific knowledge but was also able to readily use lay language effectively.

This scene also illustrates why there is a temptation, and tendency, for nurses to remain in the security of their "guild", with its secret knowledge, passed down from person-to-person, from nurse-to-nurse, via the apprentice model, because this offers the rewards of a rich, connected and supportive community. Yet, such inward-looking practice also condemns nurses to a future where nursing knowledge stagnates, is not shared, and the profession cannot rise in public recognition or esteem.

Nursing knowledges in action

The 2018 bestselling autobiographical memoir, *The Language of Kindness*, chronicles the twenty years Christie Watson worked as a Registered Nurse in Britain's National Health Service. Highly skilled, Watson has practiced in contexts ranging from mental health to paediatric intensive care, and has been appointed to highly responsible positions such as team leader of the resuscitation team for a busy London hospital. In her book, Watson recounts her fears and mistakes, as well as satisfactions and joys. For her, nursing is defined by acts of care, compassion and kindness. Her account also embodies highly developed nursing knowledges, demonstrating scientific expertise, as well as a humane and humble standpoint that together constitute the essence of nursing.

She describes how a two-year-old girl, Charlotte, with "a high temperature, a high heart rate and a few tiny purple spots of rash" is rushed to hospital.

Although "It doesn't sound much. She is conscious and talking", Watson notes that she, and the retrieval team, understand "the nature of sepsis". One of the retrieval team, Tracy, telephones ahead noting her deteriorating condition. "She's needed so much fluid to treat her shock that her lungs are drowning in it, and she's frothing at the mouth like a rabid dog". Watson describes her arrival and initial treatment:

> She is on a trolley covered in tubes already, a ventilator at her head end and a monitor by her feet ... Tracy hands over her details while we walk, pushing the trolley to the bed space where Dusan has rolled up his already short-sleeved shirt ... It is impossible to cannulate her, as her veins are too difficult to find. I position her leg in front of me – it is cold and pale, like a twig from a dying tree – and screw an intraosseous needle into her bone, confirming placement with the sudden crunch ... The purple rash has spread.
>
> (2018, pp. 237–238)

She is realistic about the little girl's chances:

> I know when I hand over, long after my shift should have ended, that it is unlikely Charlotte will be there in the morning; that she'll need three nurses at a minimum just to care for her, and she'll probably lose her almost completely dead and purple legs, and possibly her arms too.
>
> (p. 238)

At the same time, she is concerned about the other nurses and their reactions:

> I look at the nurse taking over from me, who will likely hold Charlotte's leg as it is cut off on the ward. She is fairly junior and already this week has had to pull a mother off a child who died, the mother trying desperately to give him chest compressions after the team had stopped. She has taken another mother to the mortuary.
>
> (2018, p. 239)

She continues, comparing the nurses' and doctors' roles:

> What is the cost of all this to the nurses, I wonder, and how little is it valued? The surgeon will come and remove Charlotte's leg. Then leave. The amazing paediatric intensive-care doctors will spend ten minutes explaining what needed to be done, and why, to the family. Then leave. The nurse will hold Charlotte's leg as it is being cut off. Then she will sit with Charlotte's parents for ten or twelve hours, through the entire night, watching over Charlotte.
>
> (2018, pp. 239–240)

Nurses are, therefore, by default, the parents' main information source:

> Performing her nursing tasks, as they ask her a million questions that they felt unable to ask the doctors: Is she in pain? Will she walk? Will she live? Can she hear me? Why did this happen to her? What does it mean? Do you think she will make it? Is she dying?
>
> (2018, p. 240)

In this account, Watson demonstrates a highly developed nursing world view in which she draws upon empirical and experiential knowledge. She has clearly seen this kind of sepsis in a child before and can anticipate the likely sequelae should the child be treated too late, or not respond to treatment. She also feels empathy for Charlotte and for the nurse taking over and thus displays what Carper (1978) describes as personal knowledge. Her consideration of what the parents are going through, with the questions that they might be needing to ask, the decisions that may be imminent is an indication of a moral stance and ethical knowing.

Another example of the caring role requiring additional, or even alternative, bases of knowledge to the scientific is found in another memoir, Tilda Shalof's *A Nurse's Story* (2005). Recounting her time as an intensive care nurse in Canada, Shalof's narrative contains traces of the good nurse and what has been described as "the virtue script". As Gordon and Nelson (2006) explain, the good nurse stereotype is so widely known within society, that it comes to nursing students already available, as if it is a pre-written script. This script directs nurses to be demure, selfless and kind, and for patients and others to respond warmly to them when these virtues are displayed. When they are not, nurses doubt themselves, even though the script is ill-fitting and out-dated. Shalof details instances in which she was trying to be all-caring but ran out of energy or lacked the skills required, and others where she had to engage in actions that could not be thought of as "good" nursing. Her narrative also shows that sometimes it is necessary to be empathic but at others, both for the good of the patient and/or in the interests of the nurse's own self-care, it is necessary to "turn off" and be less engaged. In this way, *A Nurse's Story* describes an unseen aspect of the nurse's role: how nurses have to make far-reaching decisions about when to act or not, and – as Watson suggests – how they then need to draw boundaries around the stresses of work so that they can resume normal home lives. In one scene, Nurse Tilda speaks to another ICU nurse about a critically ill patient:

> "... do you really think it's going to be tonight?" [the other nurse asks].
>
> "I have a feeling." I have learned to trust my feelings ... Sometimes we call a family meeting to discuss the death and how we will let it happen ... We convene in a shabby, cramped room called the "quiet room". It is a tiny room with buzzing fluorescent lights, no windows ... The quiet

room! It is probably the most disquieting place in the whole hospital. Bombs are detonated in here.

"... if we were to let him go," she asks me ... "What would the cause of death be?"

"... multi-system organ failure." I take a breath before the list of Mr De Witt's medical problems: "Overwhelming sepsis, disseminated intravascular coagulation, pancreatitis, renal failure, and complications of diabetes".

"Oh" [the other nurse replies].

(2005, pp. 2–8)

This snapshot from one nurse-nurse encounter during a busy ICU shift conveys the depth of emotional labour involved in nursing and the kinds of skills nurses require to understand, explore and control their own emotions as well as the feelings of others. In this encounter, Shalof is not only aware of the way in which intuition can influence the situation, she also makes decisions about whether or not to trust this non-reasoning process. Ultimately, she does place her trust in her feelings, for her past experience has taught her that these count. This mirrors a more complex theory put forward by Benner (2000) about the ways in which expert nurses access multiple data sources, including those which are empirically measurable, and others which are more implicit and subtle, in order to swiftly and effectively make clinical judgements. In addition, the passage portrays how such nurses may rehearse communication options before taking action. As a competent nurse, Shalof reveals how she will attempt to manage both her own emotions and those of the family and dispense only the information required under the circumstances. Such advanced emotional intelligence requires dexterity and sensitivity. In this exchange, as in many other scenes, Shalof's narrative reveals her to be a knowledge-worker utilising both intuitive, and rational scientific, understandings. She also shows that she has a deep understanding that her work as a nurse encompasses delivering both highly technical care and emotional comfort to her patients and their families, as well as other nurses when necessary.

After this evening shift, Shalof completes the necessary paperwork, and returns home to her partner. When he asks her, "How was work?", she replies, "Fine, no problem." When he asks if it was busy, she replies, "Yes", and notes, "And we leave it at that." But she continues to think about the shift:

Should I tell him the truth? That I helped a man die, that I comforted his wife who sobbed in my arms, and that no, I am not upset about it. This is what I do for a living as a nurse in the intensive care unit.

(p. 12)

This brief passage of dialogue and the nurse's reflection upon it suggests that something far more subtle and expert than scientific knowledge is required, and drawn upon, by intensive care nurses completing their everyday work. Apart from empathising with the patient, Shalof suggests that nursing requires resilience, courage and strength of mind as well as a sense of what is required in terms of self-preservation when assisting others. Shalof writes that "Nursing is the opposite of despair; it offers the opportunity to do something about suffering", but notes the various strengths that are required in order to do so. She continues:

> you have to be strong to be a nurse. You need strong muscles and stamina for the long shifts and heavy lifting, intelligence and discipline to acquire knowledge and exercise critical thinking. As for emotional fortitude – well, I'm still working on that. Most of all, you need moral courage because nursing is about the pursuit of justice. It requires you stand up to bullies, to do things that are right but difficult, and to speak your mind even when you are afraid. I wasn't strong like this when I started out. Nursing made me strong.
>
> (Back cover)

The nursing qualities that Shalof displays and describes in her matter-of fact prose – these strengths; stamina; intelligence; the discipline to acquire knowledge and exercise critical thinking; emotional fortitude, moral courage and a willingness to pursue justice, to stand up to bullies, to do things that are right but difficult, and to speak her mind even when she was afraid of the consequences – are all qualities that, if questioned, most patients would attest to wanting in the nurses entrusted with their care. They are certainly those which are currently discussed as being of supreme value in light of scandals of nursing neglect (Francis, 2013; Sawbridge and Hewison, 2011).

Conclusion

Three centuries ago, community healers who did not fit the strict criteria set down for medical practitioners – to be male, studying medicine, Plato, Aristotle and Christian doctrine – were suppressed, rejected and exiled. The knowledge that healers developed was derided and looked upon suspiciously and yet patients came to them, asking – and grateful for – the specialised help they offered, even though the rationales behind their remedies were enigmatic. Today, narratives in popular culture vividly illustrate that important aspects of nursing knowledge remain beyond scientific reasoning, and involve intuition, emotion, compassion and kindness. Such recognition tends to lead, however, to the dismissal of this kind of unscientific knowledge as "soft" and belonging to the realm of the traditional feminine. Use of this knowledge can also lead to the actions of (at least some) nurses being regarded with suspicion and being perceived as a threat to the social order. Yet, such knowledge systems, which are difficult to articulate and often unable to be quantified or tested are, paradoxically, a potential power source for nurses because they enhance not only the nurse's effectiveness but contribute to a unique nursing identity.

Reference

Austgard K (2006) The aesthetic experience of nursing *Nursing Philosophy* 7: 11–19.

Benner P (2000) The wisdom of our practice. *AJN The American Journal of Nursing* 100(10): 99–105.

Briggs R (1996) *Witches & Neighbours: The Social and Cultural Context of European Witchcraft.* New York: Viking.

Carlile M (2013) Whatever happened to the art of nursing? Available at: www.death talker.com/whatever-happened-to-the-art-of-nursing.

Carper B (1978) Fundamental patterns of knowing in nursing *Advances in Nursing Science* 1(1): 13–24.

Charon R (2008) *Narrative Medicine: Honoring the Stories of Illness.* Oxford: Oxford University Press.

Cuthbert A (2003) *The Oxford Companion to the Body.* Oxford: Oxford University Press.

Donahue M (1985) Nursing: The finest art, an illustrated history *The American Journal of Nursing* 85(12): 1352.

Donelan K, Buerhaus P, DesRoches C, Dittus R and Dutwin D (2008) Public perceptions of nursing careers: The influence of the media and nursing shortages *Nursing Economics* 26(3): 143.

Dossey B M, Keegan L and Guzzetta C E (2005) *Holistic Nursing: A Handbook for Practice* (4th ed.). Sudbury, MA: Jones and Bartlett Publishers.

Edwards S (1998) The art of nursing *Nursing Ethics* 5(5): 393–400.

Ehrenreich B and English D (2010) *Witches, Midwives, & Nurses: A History of Women Healers.* New York: The Feminist Press.

Eriksson K (2002) Caring science in a new key *Nursing Science Quarterly* 15(1): 61–65.

Francis R (2013) *Independent Inquiry into Care Provided by Mid-Staffordshire NHS Foundation Trust, 2005–2009.* Surrey: Office of Public Sector Information.

Gadamer H (2004) *The Enigma of Health.* Oxford: Blackwell.

Gordon S and Nelson S (2006) Moving beyond the virtue script in nursing: Creating a knowledge-based identity for nurses. Nelson S and Gordon S (eds) *The Complexities of Care: Nursing Reconsidered.* New York: Cornell University Press, 13–29.

Green M (2006) Getting to the source: The case of Jacoba Felicie and the impact *Medieval Feminist Forum* 42: 49–62.

Hegge M (2011) The lingering presence of the Nightingale legacy *Nursing Science Quarterly* 24(2): 152–162.

Jenner C (1997) The art of nursing: A concept analysis *Nursing Forum* 32(4): 5–11.

Johns C (1995) Framing learning through reflection within Carper's fundamental ways of knowing in nursing *Journal of Advanced Nursing* 22(2): 226–234.

Kalanithi P (2016) *When Breath Becomes Air.* New York: Random House.

Martin D (dir) (2016) Episode 7. *Call the Midwife.* Series 5. Television series. London: Neal Street Productions.

McCormack B and McCance T (2011) *Person-centred Nursing: Theory and Practice.* New York: John Wiley & Sons.

Morris-Thompson T, Shepherd J, Plata R and Marks-Maran D (2011) Diversity, fulfilment and privilege: The image of nursing *Journal of Nursing Management* 19(5): 683–692.

Mullangi S (2013) The synergy of medicine and art in the curriculum *Academic Medicine* 88(7): 921–923.

Nichols D (dir) (1946) *Sister Kenny.* Film. Hollywood: RKO Pictures.

Nightingale F (1860) *Notes on Nursing: What It Is and What It Is Not*. London: Harrison.

O'Brien C (2008) *Never Say Die*. Sydney: HarperCollins.

Ozaras G and Abaan S (2016) Investigation of the trust status of the nurse–patient relationship *Nursing Ethics* 25(5): 628–639.

Pearson H (2013) Science and intuition: Do both have a place in clinical decision making? *British Journal of Nursing* 22(4): 212–215.

Petty N, Cross V and Stew G (2012) Professional doctorate level study: The experience of health professional practitioners in their first year *Work Based Learning e-Journal* 2(2): Available at: http://wblearning-ejournal.com/archive/10-03–12

Moore RD (2014–current) *Outlander*. Television series. Culver City: Sony Pictures Television.

Ross P (1983) Kenny E 1880–1952 *Australian Dictionary of Biography*. Canberra: National Centre of Biography, Australian National University.

Sawbridge Y and Hewison A (2011) *Time to Care? Responding to Concerns about Poor Nursing Care*. Birmingham: University of Birmingham.

Shafer A (2017) *Healing Arts: The Synergy of Medicine and the Humanities*. Palo Alto: Stanford Medicine.

Shalof T (2005) *A Nurse's Story*. New York: Random House.

Thomas H (creator) (2012–current) *Call the Midwife*. Television series. London: Neal Street Productions.

Wainwright P (2000) Towards an aesthetics of nursing *Journal of Advanced Nursing* 32(3): 750–755.

Watson C (2018) *The Language of Kindness: A Nurse's Story*. London: Chatto & Windus.

White J (1995) Patterns of knowing: Review, critique, and update *Advances in Nursing Science* 17(4): 73–86.

Wicks D (1998) *Nurses and Doctors at Work: Rethinking Professional Boundaries*. Buckingham: Open University Press.

Worth J (2002) *Call the Midwife*. London: Merton Books.

Worth J (2005) *Shadows of the Workhouse*. London: Weidenfeld & Nicholson.

Worth J (2009) *Farewell to the East End*. London: Orion Publishing Company.

3   Objects of desire

Introduction

The English film *Carry on Doctor* (Thomas, 1967) begins with a long take of a nurse (played by Barbara Windsor) walking or, rather, *sashaying* to Eric Rogers' bouncy orchestral soundtrack, from one hospital building to another. She wears a short pink uniform, covered with a white apron, seamed black stockings and high heels, her brassy blonde hair tied up in a messy bun under a white cap. Along her walk she passes several male admirers – a cyclist sounds his bell at her, a chauffeur bellows, "What about *that* then!", and a man fixing a car responds with a loud exclaim, "phwoah!". The nurse giggles and blows them a kiss.

The sexualisation of nursing's image is long-standing, with the "naughty nurse" trope familiar and widespread. It is, indeed, difficult to think of another profession that is so closely linked to such sexist discourse. Such sexualised imagery of the nurse in popular culture set up expectations for how people approach interactions with nurses, in the process shaping public understanding about nurses and the nursing profession. At worst, nurses are sex objects in these depictions while, at best, they humanise and lighten the atmosphere of a hospital context that would otherwise conjure ideas of rigidity, control, order and fear. In these ways, the depiction of a nurse as sexually desirable and available is paradoxical because on the one hand, the notion is unrealistic and sexist, but on the other, nursing's connection to desire is intriguing. Hearn (2013, p. 54) also notes, that many of these jokes are motivated by anxiety and fear of a loss of dignity and, thus, it can be no accident that so many of these representations feature nurses, nursing and health care. In this reading, such imagery is a manifestation of projected anxiety about being hospitalised and cared for intimately by strangers.

Smith's (1987) work in critical social science suggests that exploring the realm of the everyday for examples where power relations and conventional ways of thinking give an object its meaning is an important exercise as such an analysis can reveal how that object is constrained and marginalised. In this case, teasing out the image of the "naughty nurse" can assist in revealing contradictions and ambiguities about nursing's public image. The sexualisation of nursing is reductive, patronising and sexist – tools consciously or unconsciously used by a prevailing and conservative dominant paradigm to maintain social order and prevent change (Hallam, 2012). Within health, this may mean preserving policies and practices that are medically driven and in which nurses can only play a subordinate role. Continued imaging of nurses in this reduced way maintains a narrative that no longer holds (if it ever did hold), but helps to explain why nursing continues to struggle for status, including leadership status, within health policy and practice. Yet, in contradiction, this perception of nursing also has a glamourous aspect and this glamour has a positive side. For storytellers, for instance, having an attractive, willing and able nurse character to support action within a plot, provides for viewing pleasure (Mulvey, 1989). Not only is the audience satisfied, but this, in turn, cements nursing's positive (though limited) profile within the minds of the viewing public.

Sexy nurses

Much of the comedy in the bawdy series of English *Carry On* films (1958–1978, 1992) that are set in hospitals – with *Carry On Nurse* (Thomas, 1959), *Carry On Again Doctor* (Thomas, 1969) and *Carry On Matron* (Thomas, 1972), alongside the example of *Carry On Doctor* (discussed above) – involves the nursing staff in such scenarios. Well-known for their slapstick, farcical plots, and vaudevillian characterisation and delivery, the *Carry On* films are (in)famous for their double entendre and sexual innuendo. Many of the nurses in these films are portrayed as attractive, obedient, efficient and servile – conforming, therefore, to the stereotype of "angels with pretty faces" (Darbyshire, 2010). Unlike, however, the idealised "good nurse" who is demure and modest, *Carry On* nurses have bright, alluring smiles and shapely, ample figures that threaten to burst out of the tight uniforms in which they are barely contained. Much general hilarity arises from the convoluted antics involved in keeping the various professional and personal (including romantic and potentially sexual) "goings-on" and transgressions from the authority figure of the matron. The viewers for whom these scripts were written were not expecting realism, but wanted to laugh at jokes that were written in contravention of what would be later defined as political correctness.

The films are – according to Chapman (2012) – "a cherished and much-loved national institution" (p. 100) for their unapologetic vulgarity and their irreverent spoofing of otherwise respected institutions and customs, and rejection of "authority and respectability" (2012, p. 100), although they have also long been criticised for their coarse crudity (Gerrard, 2016). When they were produced, such depictions would be read by most as light-hearted fun. Today, of course, they are understood to be sexist and demeaning. The portrayal of nurses in these films is not unlike the way they are depicted in the British comic cartoon seaside postcard. These postcards have been, and continue to be, variously described as "ribald", "saucy", "cheeky" and "naughty" by their appreciators, while critics describe these examples of an identifiably British form of humour as "prurient", "lurid", "vulgar", "blatant", "in bad taste", "offensive", "indecent" and, even, "obscene". The longevity and commercial success of these cards (which has stretched from the Edwardian era until today) has been linked to ideas of a seaside holiday as one of liberty, hedonism and sexual licentiousness (Gray, 2006, p. 86; Stratiev, 2009, p.193). While most of these suggestive, salacious and usually sexist comic cartoons – comprising a drawing accompanied by a text punch-line – are set on the beach, pier or foreshore, a subset feature hospitals. Like the *Carry On* films, the jokes featured on these cards rely heavily on phallic imagery and innuendo, referring to male bodies and penises being inadvertently fondled or damaged, or patient-nurse sexual contact. Also in common with the *Carry On* films, the matrons in these cartoons are usually portrayed as cross, heavy and older, while the nurses are younger and attractively curvaceous. The nurses are also often portrayed as sexually naïve, while the matrons are all-knowing.

The sexual fantasies inspired by mass produced pin-up and calendar girls, popular with male soldiers in war to divert their attention from the reality at hand and as encouraged by government bureaucracies as morale boosters (Kakoudaki, 2004), has been a major and successful plot line for military-medical dramas. This can be seen in the high rating television comedy-drama series M*A*S*H (Gelbart and Reynolds, 1972–1983). Set in South Korea during the Korean War, the series was based on the fictional *MASH: A Novel About Three Army Doctors* by Richard Hooker (1968). Among the key personnel of the US army mobile surgical hospital that gave the series its title, Head Nurse Major Margaret Houlihan (played by Loretta Swit) appeared regularly

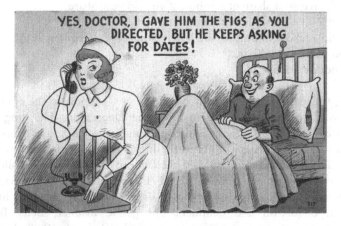

Figure 3.1 A comic cartoon postcard ca. 1930s, now considered sexist and as objectifying nurses.

in all eleven seasons of the programme. Often just called "Margaret", and nicknamed "Hot lips" Houlihan both for her sexy attractiveness and her fiery, passionate nature, this nurse was the highest-ranking female officer in the unit. Despite this rank, or perhaps because of it, Houlihan functions as a figure of romantic interest for many of the men in the male-dominated environment. She is the focus of much innuendo and less veiled sexually-focused comment, some of this directed to the way she fills out her regulation uniform, and she also serves as foil for many of the men's jokes. It is noteworthy that all the nurses in this long-running television series, including Houlihan, were depicted wearing army greens, but the shapeless uniforms were refashioned to emphasise their wearers' desirability. As the child of army personnel, she is a stickler for rules, although she has a long affair with married surgeon Frank Burns. Despite this sexualisation, Hoolihan was also shown to be a competent leader, guiding and organising the women nurses who were serving in the unit under her command (Buchanan, 1997).

When dressed in a nursing uniform and delivering care to a ward of sick patients, the cartoon figure of Betty Boop is an early example of sexualised imaging at work. Betty Boop was a popular animated character created by Max Fleisher in the 1930s, featuring in cartoons that played in movie theatres around the world (Fleischer, 2005). In *A Song a Day* (Fleischer, 1936), Betty plays a nurse who tends to a hospital ward filled with animal patients. Wearing a tight white uniform, cute cap, signature hoop earrings and heavy make-up, Betty is attentive and loving in her administrations. She sings a song as she happily goes about her work:

> Your life will be worth living if you do your share
> You'll find a thrill in giving that's beyond compare
> An understanding touch, a sympathetic word
> Can drive away those troubles like the song of a bird
> You'll have your share of sunshine if you do your share
> Spread a little sunshine here and there
> To help a fellow in distress you'll help yourself to happiness
> If you just do your share.
> Boo boopy doop!

The song was designed to persuade people to give support to the community in what was, at the time, mired in the Great Depression. The song advises audiences to be generous, giving and community-minded, just as Nurse Betty is. In this way, the narrative positions the nurse as a model for selfless nurture and care. Double-entendres are used throughout the cartoon, signalling that Betty is available to meet many needs. Importantly, in being desired by others, Nurse Betty also finds happiness. With her round baby-face, little-girl voice, and coquettish and confident but gentle manner, Betty Boop is regarded as one of the first screen sex symbols (Barboza, 1988), her figure emphasised by tight cleavage-revealing bodices and high heels. Her familiar image endures, continuing to be used on a wide range of merchandise and many Betty Boop cartoons available for purchase and viewing on the internet.

In *A Song a Day*, Betty Boop is at once naïve and sexy – a paradox that is perhaps metonymic for the contemporary sexualised nursing image. One aspect of what is alluring about the "sexy nurse" is that she is unknowing of the secret desires of those who observe her, intending only to be helpful, but also unable to hide her youthful, healthy attractiveness. Fagin and Diers (1983) argue the nurse-as-sex-object metaphor stems from the idea that nurses have intimate contact with patients' bodies; that, having "seen and touched the bodies of strangers, nurses are perceived as willing and able sexual partners" (p. 116). Ironically, in politically incorrect comedy, and in pornography, the proudly held nursing values of providing intimate care, as well as being accessible, nurturing (Griffiths et al., 2012) and non-judgemental (Iacono, 2007), are corrupted in ways that denigrate and demean nursing (Summers and Summers, 2014).

Objectification of the nurse

Objectification, the act of treating a person like an object or thing (Langton, 2009; Nussbaum, 1995) is apparent in a scene from "The Contest" (Cherones, 1992) episode from the *Seinfeld* television series (1989–1998) that comedically exploits the image of the nurse. The four friends (Elaine, Jerry, Kramer and George) are bemoaning their relationship difficulties and decide to bet on who can delay the urge to masturbate the longest. George is feeling confident of winning the contest because he has to visit his mother in hospital and is sure it will be a boring experience. At the hospital, George visits Mrs. Costanza, who is propped up in a bed surrounded by closed curtains. They begin their usual critical banter and, in the middle of arguing about George's personal and professional incompetence, the screens to the patient next door are heard being pulled open. George catches a glimpse of an attractive young nurse about to attend to her patient, saying, "Hi Denise. It's six-thirty. Time for your sponge bath." The patient wakes slowly and asks lazily, "Six thirty? Is it that time already?" George's interest is piqued as this "girl-on-girl", nurse-patient encounter is, for him, an ultimate fantasy. While his parents continue their bickering, the lights dim and the screen to Denise's bed is backlit, allowing the bathing ritual to be visible in silhouette to George. He hears the nurse say, "Here. Let me help you off with that. Slip it over your head". George is now in an excruciatingly uncomfortable situation – visiting his annoying mother and having his one chance to be a voyeur to a nurse-patient sexual encounter stymied. As usual, George loses out – he neither gets to watch, nor win the contest.

This narrative representation of a nurse draws on the ancient feminine archetypes of woman as lover and mother. As lover, the nurse is naturally seductive, inciting arousal and passion in others. As mother, she is inclined to take care of others, putting their needs ahead of her own (Wolff, 1956). The first laugh is when George sees the silhouettes, and the viewer watches him watching the private act, a double pleasure. The audience knows that this is a temptation for George – not only is this a young, nubile, uniform-wearing nurse tending carefully to the body of another, but that patient is female, another forbidden pleasure. It seems unlikely that George will be able to resist this pleasure and, finally, he is almost, but not quite, caught in this act of voyeurism. Because the nurse's body and sexual appeal are emphasised, rather than her identity, at least six properties of objectification are apparent within this scene. These are: instrumentality (treating the person as a tool for another's purposes), fungibility (treating the person as interchangeable with (other) objects), violability (treating the person as lacking in boundary integrity), denial of subjectivity (treating the person as though there is no need for concern for their experiences or feelings), reduction to the body (identifying the person with their body, or body parts) and, reduction to appearance (treating a person primarily in terms of how they look or appear to the senses) (Langton, 2009; Nussbaum, 1995). The private interaction between the nurse and female patient is not respected, and George secretly watches them for his own pleasure, without anyone (including his mother, the patient or the nurse) being aware or giving consent. His desire to be titillated is more important than any other person's rights or needs.

Seinfeld was a comedy success due to its formula of amplifying and deconstructing everyday cultural practices, cleverly turning commonplace aspects of everyday life into jokes (Double, 2014). This scene is amusing because the audience is watching a trickster (George) subvert conventions of how one should act in such a situation. It also amplifies and ridicules entrenched patterns of sexism, and the sexual fetishisation of nurses. George, playing the fool, transgresses every social rule between male and female, visitor and nurse, son and mother. He tries to get away with what others in society would not be permitted to do, but ultimately his transgression is punished. Not only is his sexist behaviour thwarted, he does not win the contest either. Of interest in this scene in the context of nursing identity is the grain of truth in the scenario regarding nursing identity. Playing the fool, George, exposes a taboo in health care – that people find the very idea of the nurse "sexy". As Welsford (1961) explained, fools allow society to reflect on, and laugh at, its own complex power relations. Thus, George reveals how not to behave in the world, in the process exposing lingering and taken-for-granted aspects of power and identity in health care. The nurse is desired because, firstly, she is young and female and, secondly, because she performs caring and intimate acts of nurturing that fulfil primal Oedipal desires.

It can be conjectured that Oedipal ideas are at the root of why the nurse – as lover and mother – is a desirable and desired entity. In Greek mythology, Oedipus was a ruler who unknowingly killed his father, married his mother and suffered for this misdeed. According to Freud, an infant's first love object is its mother and childhood development involves an internal struggle where the child sees the father as a rival, fears being punished for this and learns to push this fantasy (and its attendant anxiety) into their unconscious and so develop normally as a reasoned person (Storr, 1989). Later in life, mother figures such as nurses may trigger these old fantasies, offering both a source for pleasure as well as unease. The patient no longer knows or understands why they desire the care of an ever-present, always caring nurse, but they do. In times of vulnerability and weakness such as illness or a health crisis, it may be that there is increased need for this motherly nurse. Indeed, in times of war, the figure of the nurturing nurse who is willing, able and available to perform any act of mercy deemed necessary has been used to appease distress and the fear of soldiers dying alone (Darbyshire and Gordon, 2005). Numerous propaganda posters, news stories, postcards and films were created to convey this pacifying message, providing an important counterpoint to the chaos and destruction of war.

Another clear case of objectification can be seen in Imogen Edwards-Jones' *Hospital Babylon* (2011), subtitled *True Confessions from the Front Line of Accident and Emergency*. This narrative non-fiction "exposé" purports to be completely factual. Its author writes that the hospital the story is set in is fictionalised and the action set in a 24 hour period, but everything else is true.

> Only the names have been changed ... All the anecdotes, the situations, the highs, the lows, the drugs, the excesses, the waste, the sadness and the insanity are as told to me by ... a collection of some of the finest and most successful consultants, doctors, nurses and physicians in the country.
>
> (p.8)

Yet, in this story, the only part nurses play apart from having sex with the various doctors is to whisk away and eat patients' chocolates. The nurses in this book are portrayed as always available and promiscuous.

Fetishisation and nursing

Pornography is visual material containing explicit descriptions or displays of sex, intended to stimulate erotic rather than aesthetic or emotional feelings (Seltzer, 2011). The graphic representations of pornography tend towards the explicit, grotesque and indiscriminate (McKinnon, 1995). How this demeans nursing is illustrated in explicitly sexual or pornographic films such as *I, A Woman* (Ahlberg, 1965), *Naughty Nurse* (Bartel, 1969), *Nurse-Made* (Mansfield, 1971), *Candy Stripe Nurses* (Holleb, 1974), *The Sensuous Nurse* (Rossati, 1975) and *Naughty Nurse Nancy* (DeVoe, 2009). A scene from the exploitation film *Night Call Nurses* (Kaplan, 1972) demonstrates this. Three pretty young uniformed nurses are chatting at the nurses' station, when an elderly patient approaches them. One nurse whispers to another, "Uh Oh. Bathrobe Benny is at it again!". The patient approaches, wearing only a dressing gown, and says, "Good afternoon ladies. I'm so glad to see you looking so chipper and bright on such an exquisite day!". One nurse stands and, smiling sweetly, answers, "You seem cheerful as always this morning Benny!" The camera pans back to reveal the nurse wearing a very short white dress. He responds in a seemingly polite way, "Well you know the sight of such a charming girl always gives a *lift* to an old man's spirit!", however, he then unties the robe's belt and exposes himself to her. Obviously having seen his behaviour before, the nurse is unfazed. She playfully berates his puerile behaviour and then links her arm in his, to escort him back to bed. In this film, the narrative draws on an idea of the nurse as the archetypal maiden – youthful, adventurous, fun loving and naïve – but debases her, by reducing her to nothing but a sexually available body.

The movie *Nurse 3D* (Aarniokoski, 2013) verges on the camp and grotesque. Miles (1991) explains that the grotesque, created and popularised by men for male pleasure and female humiliation, was specifically designed to debase the sexual female body, reducing it to an object of ridicule. The protagonist in *Nurse 3D*, Abby Russell (Paz de la Huerta) similarly perverts nursing work and identity in her criminal behaviour. Nurse Abby is an experienced, skilled nurse who is also very disturbed, harbouring a deep-seated desire to avenge her early childhood abandonment and barely containing her preoccupation with sex. She wears a wrap-around white uniform (suggesting that it could easily be removed) that shows her ample cleavage each time she bends to attend to a patient in bed. The shoes she wears are impractical stilettos and long strands of dark hair escape from her cap and need to be flicked away repeatedly from her heavily painted scarlet lips. Abby befriends female nursing colleagues and then seduces and abandons them. She soon moves on to doctors in the hospital – particularly those she knows have been unfaithful to their spouses. They too are seduced, but then tortured with surgical instruments before being murdered in various bloody ways. The film takes the stereotype which represents nurses as sexually primal and out of control (Ferns and Chojnacka, 2005) to an extreme, suggesting that nurses have chosen to work in health care simply to exercise their lascivious desires.

The white-dress uniform that most of these nurses wear contributes to this sense of debasement. After the Second World War, the white dress became ubiquitous for nurses. With the use of synthetic fabric making it wash-and-wear (Houweling, 2004), it was a symbol of cleanliness and sterility that functioned as an "armour of probity and purity" (Barber, 1997, p. 27) and provided an assurance of safety. From the 1970s, however, nurses began to reject dress codes that patronised or sexualised them, and when anti-discrimination laws were enacted, female nurses were allowed to wear pantsuits (Stokowski, 2017). Mass produced scrubs (a unisex pants-and-top cotton ensemble) have become the norm, and have begun to be shown in television series such as *ER* (2003–2011) and *Scrubs* (2001–2010). The white uniform remains common however in popular culture representations of nurses. This can be seen, for example, in comedies such as *Inside*

Amy Schumer (McFaul, 2014), in dramas when nursing's purity is being sat-irised such as in *The Dark Knight* (Nolan, 2008) and *Cloud Atlas* (Wachowski, Tykwer and Wachowski, 2012), adult reality television pro-gramming such as *Scrubbing In* (Osper et al., 2013–current), and hospital-inspired computer games such as *Sanitarium* (1998–current). In many of these examples, the dress is also worn shorter and tighter than what would be practical, or how it was worn when it was the usual uniform. The ongoing use of the white dress uniform as a signifier for nursing reveals how anachronistic ideas about nursing can be perpetuated and influence public ideas and misconceptions about nursing (Brien and McAllister, 2019).

The nurse's uniform can also function as a fetishised object in a wide range of popular culture products and productions, including in costume-themed events such as Halloween (Macmillan, Lynch and Bradley, 2011) and costumed sexual role play, known as cosplay. In these instances, the uniform, which is generally understood to stand for innocence and purity, is defiled and, because it is used to signify the nurse, the nurse's role is reduced, and the person referred to is dehumanised (Hallam, 2012). In more graphic objectifications of the nurse, the uniform is stretched, ripped and unbuttoned, revealing lacy bras, suspenders and stockings, and the white cap is placed at an alluring angle on long hair. Worn in this manner, the uniform becomes a sign of the nurse's availability as sexual object. The eroticisation of a nurse's image typically includes subjugation, domination, or other abuses of power. *Peep Show* (Redhead, 2004), the first novel in a popular series by Leigh Redhead, features Simone Kirsch, a stripper who leaves the sex industry to become a private investigator. The novel features strippers and lap dancers in white dresses and caps, a key plot point being the point that sex workers know this is a common male fantasy.

As Buchanan (1997) argues, this often-repeated stereotype of the nurse as sex object is not innocuous, for it ridicules nursing work and suggests that nursing is, itself, an excuse for women to play with men – from teas-ing, sexually exploiting to sado-masochistically torturing them. Power plays a role in sexualisation and objectification and, as described in Chapter 2, the use and abuse of power plays an important part in nursing's history. While the status and public image for nurses has lifted progressively since the nineteenth century (Hegge, 2011), nursing has also become primarily a role for women and, as a gendered profession, it has remained vulnerable to sexism and marginalisation. As well as the explicitly sexual or porno-graphic films such as those noted above, such sexualisation of nurses takes centre-stage in otherwise much more seemingly innocuous television soap operas such as *General Hospital* (1963–current) and *The Young Doctors* (1976–1983), and the romance novel, where romantic storylines involving sexual relationships between (male) doctors and (female) nurses are often central to the narrative.

Nurses' desirability

Alfred Eisenstaedt's now iconic photograph of a sailor impulsively kissing a nurse in Times Square, New York, on Victory Day 1945, was first published on the cover of *Life Magazine*. This image continues to resonate with viewers seventy-five years later. At the time, it embodied the excitement of celebrating the end of a world war. That it was a serviceman and a (female) nurse made it all the more meaningful. These two human beings were representative of groups who played a vital role in the fight for liberation. In a sense, this photograph represents the world's acknowledgement of all the soldiers who went to war and all the nurses who cared for wounded soldiers. Both displayed courage and skill. This nurse is, moreover, young, attractive and fun-loving. While this is a photograph capturing one impulsive, joyous moment in time, it is redolent of many images of nurses, including propaganda posters (McCrann, 2009). These posters and other images position nurses as attractive, available and indispensable, which, by association, present nursing as an exciting, valuable and noble career. The emphasis on the feminine qualities of nurses (even though men have been nurses for thousands of years) served a particular purpose in propaganda – to recruit male military service personnel (Smith, 2008), and this trope has persisted. By far the majority of nurses portrayed on screen and in novels is female.

In the scene described in the Introduction of this book, the innocent, eager, compassionate and attractive Nurse Tallis is called to sit with a French soldier to calm him in his dying moments. Not only does this character conform to the sexy-nurse trope, but she is also a mother figure, an embodiment of what the soldier needs. Tallis, standing in for all nurses, is determined to give the patient what he desires for she knows it will be healing and not harmful. This imagery retells the goddess myth, where feminine archetypes of mother or lover are actually a manifestation of projected anxiety and a way to manage and lessen those fears. In Greek mythology, for instance, Iris was the personification and goddess of the rainbow. She travelled with the speed of wind from one end of the world to the other, carrying messages from the gods to mortals, and feeding and comforting the gods (Grimal, 1996).

This nurturing role is reminiscent of idealised nursing. Wanting nurses in hospitals to be the embodiments of such goddesses may be a way for patients to reduce their fears of being in pain, isolated within a strange environment and being dependent on the care provided by strangers, or their trepidation about powerful women. This aspect to the sexual imaging therefore affects not only how patients see nurses, but how nurses see themselves. It therefore contributes to nursing's identity. Thus, the sexy-nurse trope is paradoxical. On the one hand it is repellent, but on the other it has a magnetism that makes nursing appealing and impossible to ignore.

Reclaiming and subverting the stereotype

Some in health care have recognised the power of the nurse as sex-object image and turned it around to serve their purposes. Kondo and Ishikawa (2018) report on the results of an experimental public health initiative that aimed to encourage people at risk of lifestyle diseases precipitated by a lack of exercise, smoking and poor diet, to make healthy changes. Knowing that the negative emotions experienced by at-risk populations tend to compound addictive behaviours, they reasoned that positive emotions and the promise of hedonistic or other pleasure may stimulate healthy behaviour changes. To test this, Kondo and Ishikawa designed a health check service and ran it for two years in Japanese pachinko (arcade game) parlours, places where socially dis-advantaged men and women tend to congregate. The staff of this service wore what are described as "mildly erotic nurse costumes" (p. 2) consisting of a white dress with short skirt and nurse's cap, and were very attentive to those presenting for the check. The study showed that, compared to a group who received the same messages delivered by people wearing white lab coats, the pachinko customers sustained a higher level of involvement in the public health intervention. The authors suggested two reasons for this. First, the attractiveness of the "nurses" led to positive affect in the participants and more willingness to listen and engage with the information they were being given. Second, the uniform itself was seen as trustworthy and, by association, so too was the information.

There are others who suggest that use of sexual imagery and portrayal of young women as sexual are not always disempowering. For some women these representations can convey messages about career choices, power, control and influence in relationships (Macmillan, Lynch and Bradley, 2011). This illustrates a paradox around desire and nursing, that nurses are objects of desire and thus experience objectification, but they can themselves also sometimes enjoy this position, because it reinforces their admired status (Bryce, Foley and Reeves, 2017).

Conclusion

The impact of the depiction of nursing as sexy is wide-ranging. On the nega-tive side, the imaging is exploitative and objectifying. Pornographic depictions emphasise the lurid and grotesque and do not add to any realistic understanding about nursing. In this way, such imaging can be seen to devitalise nursing iden-tity and perpetuate nursing's dismissal as an object of ridicule, female and merely pretending to professionalism, existing only to please a masculinist and dominating order. More nuanced, but still sexist, depictions suggest that nurses are naïve, servile and willing to please, thus locking nurses in as only marginal players within the health service context, and incapable of participating equally in decision-making and advocacy positions. Ironically, the sexual portrayals of nurses and nursing only work because nurses are seen as attractive and desirable.

The continued imaging of nurses in this reduced way maintains an outdated myth, and helps to explain why nursing continues to struggle for status as a leader within health policy and practice. The sexy-nurse trope is therefore deeply paradoxical; while it is repellent and demeaning, it also reflects how nursing has an attractive magnetism that makes nursing charismatic, compelling and impossible to ignore.

References

Aarniokoski D dir (2013) *Nurse 3D*. Film. Hollywood: Lionsgate.

Ahlberg M dir (1965) *I, A Woman*. Film. Copenhagen: Europa Film.

Barber J (1997) Uniform and nursing reform *International History of Nursing Journal* 3(1): 20–29.

Barboza D (1988) Video world is smitten by a gun-toting, tomb-raiding sex symbol *The New York Times* 19 January D3.

Bartel P (dir) (1969) *Naughty Nurse!* Film. Hacienda-Tropican-Madness. Available at: www.youtube.com/watch?v=kjdl_CzLn7k.

Bryce J, Foley E and Reeves J (2017) Conduct most becoming *Australian Nursing and Midwifery Journal* 25(6): 25.

Buchanan T (1997) Nursing our narratives: Towards a dynamic understanding of nurses in narrative tales *Nursing Inquiry* 4(2): 80–87.

Chapman J (2012) A short history of the Carry On films. In Hunter I and Porter L *British Comedy Cinema*. London: Routledge, 100–115.

Cherones T (1992) The contest. *Seinfeld*. Television series. New York: Castlerock Entertainment.

Crichton M (creator) (2003–2011) *ER*. Television series. Hollywood: Warner.

D L Brien and McAllister M (2019) Fashioning modernity, myth and the macabre: An examination of the function of nurses' uniforms on screen *The Australasian Journal of Popular Culture* 8(1): 101–118.

Darbyshire P (2010) Heroines, hookers and harridans: Exploring popular images and representations of nurses and nursing. In Daly J, Speedy S and Jackson D *Contexts of Nursing*. Sydney: Elsevier, 51–64.

Darbyshire P and Gordon S (2005) Exploring popular images and representations of nurses and nursing In Daly J, Speedy S, Jackson D, Lambert K and Lambert C (eds) *Professional Nursing: Concepts, Issues and Challenges*. New York: Springer, 69–92.

DeVoe D (dir) (2009) *Naughty Nurse Nancy*. Video Warrendale, PA: DVD Empire.

Double O (2014) Observational comedy. In Double O (ed) *Getting the Joke: The Inner Workings of Stand-Up Comedy*. 2nd ed. London: Methuen Drama, 27.

Edwards-Jones I (2011) *Hospital Babylon: True Confessions from the Front Line of Accident and Emergency*. London: Bantam Press.

Fagin C and Dears D (1983) Nursing as metaphor *New England Journal of Medicine* 309(2): 191–192.

Ferns T and Chojnacka I (2005) Angels and swingers, matrons and sinners: Nursing stereotypes *British Journal of Nursing* 14(19): 1028–1032.

Fleischer M (creator) (1936) *A Song A Day*. Cartoon. New York: Fleischer Productions.

Fleischer R (2005) *Out of the Inkwell: Max Fleischer and the Animation Revolution*. Lexington: University Press of Kentucky.

Gelbart L and Reynolds G creators (1972–1983) *M*A*S*H*. Television Series. Los Angeles: 20th Century Fox Television.

Gerrard S (2016) *The Carry On Films*. London: Pan Macmillan.

Gray F (2006) *Designing the Seaside: Architecture, Society and Nature*. London: Reaktion books.

Griffiths J, Speed S, Horne M and Keeley P (2012) "A caring professional attitude": What service users and carers seek in graduate nurses and the challenge for educators *Nurse Education Today* 32(2): 121–127.

Grimal P (1996) *Iris: The Dictionary of Classical Mythology*. London: Blackwell.

Hallam J (2012) *Nursing the Image: Media, Culture and Professional Identity*. London: Routledge.

Hearn M (2013) *Saucy Postcards: The Bamforth Collection*. London: Constable & Robinson.

Hegge M (2011) The lingering presence of the Nightingale legacy *Nursing Science Quarterly* 24(2): 152–161.

Holleb A (dir) (1974) *Candy Stripe Nurses*. Film. Hollywood: New World Pictures.

Hooker R (1968) *MASH: A Novel About Three Army Doctors*. London: Hachete.

Houweling L (2004) Image, function, and style: A history of the nursing uniform *The American Journal of Nursing* 104(4): 40–48.

Iacono M (2007) Nurses: Trusted patient advocates *Journal of Peri-Anesthesia Nursing* 22(5): 330–334.

Kakoudaki D (2004) Pinup: The secret weapon in World War II. In Williams L (ed) *Porn Studies*. Durham and London: Dale University Press, 335–369.

Kaplan J (dir) (1972) *Night Call Nurses*. Film Hollywood: New World Pictures.

Kondo N and Ishikawa Y (2018) Affective stimuli in behavioural interventions soliciting for health check-up services and the service users' socioeconomic statuses: A study at Japanese pachinko parlours *Online Journal of Epidemiological Community Health* 72 (5). Available at https://jech.bmj.com/content/72/5/e1.

Langton R (2009) *Sexual Solipsism: Philosophical Essays on Pornography and Objectification*. Oxford: Oxford University Press.

Lawrence B (creator) (2001–2010) *Scrubs*. Television series. Hollywood: Disney.

Macmillan C, Lynch A and Bradley L (2011) Agonic and hedonic power: The performance of gender by young adults on Halloween *Paideusis: Journal for Interdisciplinary and Cross-Cultural Studies* 5: E1–30.

Mansfield R dir (1971) *Nurse-Made*. Film. New York: Mansfield Films.

McCrann G (2009) Government wartime propaganda posters: Communicators of public policy *Behavioral & Social Sciences Librarian* 28(1–2): 53–73.

McFaul I (2014) *Inside Amy Schumer – The Nurses*. Television series. Hollywood: Jax Media.

McKinnon C (1995) Speech, equality, and harm: The case against pornography In Lederer L and Delgado R (eds) *The Price We Pay: The Case against Racist Speech, Hate Propaganda, and Pornography*. New York: Hill and Wang, 301–330.

Miles M R (1991) *Carnal Knowing: Female Nakedness and Religious Meaning in the Christian West*. New York: Vintage.

Mulvey L (1989) Visual pleasure and narrative cinema In Mulvey L (ed) *Visual and Other Pleasures*. London: Palgrave Macmillan, 14–26.

Nolan C (dir) (2008) *The Dark Knight*. Film Hollywood: Warner Brothers.

Nussbaum M (1995) Objectification *Philosophy & Public Affairs* 24(4): 249–291.

Osper D, Rodgers J, Cronin M and Fitzgerald S (exec prods) (2013–current) *Scrubbing In*. Television series. Vol. 51 Hollywood: Minds Entertainment.

Price S and McGillis Hall L (2014) The history of nurse imagery and the implications for recruitment: A discussion paper *Journal of Advanced Nursing* 70(7): 1502–1509.

Redhead L (2004) *Peep Show*. Sydney: Allen & Unwin.

Rossati N dir (1975) *The Sensuous Nurse*. Film Rome: Compagnia Films.

Seltzer L (2011) What distinguishes erotica from pornography? *Psychology Today* 6 April. Available at www.psychologytoday.com/intl/blog/evolution-the-self/201104/what-distinguishes-erotica-pornography.

Smith A (2008) The girl behind the man behind the gun: Women as carers in recruitment posters of the First World War *Journal of War & Culture Studies* 1(3): 223–241.

Smith D (1987) *The Everyday World as Problematic: A Feminist Sociology*. Toronto: University of Toronto Press.

Stokowski L (2017) Nurse uniforms: Who cares what nurses wear? *Medscape Nursing Perspectives* 6 April. Available at www.medscape.com/viewarticle/878174.

Storr A (1989) *Freud: A Very Short Introduction*. Oxford: Oxford University Press.

Stratiev S (2009) The margin of the printable: Seaside postcards and censorship In Feigel L and Harris A (eds) *Modernism on Sea: Art and Culture at the British Seaside*. Oxford: Peter Lang, 191–210.

Summers S and Summers H (2014) *Saving Lives: Why the Media's Portrayal of Nursing Puts Us All at Risk*. New York: Oxford University Press.

Thomas G (dir) (1959) *Carry on Nurse*. Film. Buckinghamshire: Beaconsfield Productions.

Thomas G dir (1967) *Carry on Doctor*. Film. Buckinghamshire: Beaconsfield Productions.

Thomas G dir (1969) *Carry on Again Doctor*. Film. London: Rank Organisation.

Thomas G dir (1972) *Carry on Matron*. Film. London: Rank Organisation.

Wachowski L, Tykwer T and Wachowski A (dirs) (2012) *Cloud Atlas*. Film. Hollywood: Warner Brothers.

Welsford E (1961) *The Fool: His Social and Literary History*. New York: Doubleday.

Wolff T (1956) *Structural Forms of the Feminine Psyche*. Zurich: CG Jung Institute.

4   Nursing and the abject

Introduction

The previous chapter discussed the ways in which nursing is often presented as a glamorous profession that involves the (seemingly) easy and natural work of dispensing ordinary human kindness to patients. In Betty Boop's sweetly innocent song, this sanitised view of nursing is invoked:

> An understanding touch, a sympathetic word
> Can drive away those troubles like the song of a bird
> You'll have your share of sunshine if you do your share
> Spread a little sunshine here and there
>
> (Fleischer, 1936)

In contrast, a poignant scene from a more contemporary representation of nursing reveals another dimension to the work undertaken by nurses. It comes from an episode titled "Yesterday's News" (Roden, 1998) from the long running Australian medical drama *All Saints* (Lee, 1998–2009). Registered Nurse Jared Levine (played by Ben Tari) stands in a shower cubicle wearing a white plastic apron over his uniform. Knee-length galoshes and rubber gloves protect his feet and hands. Resigning himself to showering a dishevelled, middle-aged and filthy homeless man, Nurse Jared says – as much to himself as the man – "Okay, let's do it". There is little enthusiasm in his manner, but then he looks up and notices that his patient is also hesitant. Impatiently, Jared declares, "Well, come on! It's not that bad! I'll give you a good scrub and you'll feel much better in no time". Wordlessly, the man unbuttons his shirt, releasing a putrid smell and exposing caked-on grime and open sores. Gagging, Jared coughs out another direction: "Remove your singlet too. Let's get rid of all this and I'll get you some clean clothes". Then, trying to ease the embarrassment they both feel, he adds, "It will be better than this lot, hey?" Submissively, the patient lifts the final layer of clothing over his head, to reveal a thick layer of damp and rotting newspapers stuck to his chest. Jared is overwhelmed, barely managing to whisper out an apology before fleeing from the room to vomit.

Although this is a fictional drama, such scenes are not uncommon in the modern health care system, when nurses are required to perform close, intimate body care for people who have been living in squalid conditions due to neglect or disability. This brief scene reveals two important realities. The first is that filth and other deeply unpleasant aspects of illness, injury, disease and death are regularly encountered by health care workers. And, second, these workers are themselves not immune from what are deeply innate human reactions of disgust and horror to this aspect of nursing work. Such work lies in the realm of the abject, which as Dave Holmes, Amelie Perron and Patrick O'Byrne (2006) explain in a rare scholarly discussion of the issue, all nurses must confront. They detail how "Cadaverous, sick, disabled bodies, troubled minds, wounds, vomit, feces, and so forth are all part of nursing work and threaten the clean and proper bodies of nurses" and also note that this "unclean side of nursing is rarely accounted for in academic literature: it is silenced" (p. 305).

However, while the concept of abjection is a relatively new concept in discourse around nursing, nurses have long struggled with its presence in their daily work. Indeed, according to Susan Reverby's (1987) history of modern nursing in the United States, hospitals encountered difficulties recruiting women suited to the role at the turn of the twentieth century due to this fact. She recites the story of a nurse who told a Boston reporter in 1907 of the mismatch between the idea of nursing work, and the reality: "A woman would be better advised to take up teaching or stenography. Nursing is not what it's cracked up to be" (p. 90).

The reality is that the nursing role involves being able to both put aside one's own instincts of disgust *and* ease the patient's anxieties – a dual action that students rarely learn about (Allan et al., 2016). When nurses fail in this challenge, they may leave the patient feeling poorly understood and comforted, and their dignity may not be maintained (Doyle, Hungerford and Cruickshank, 2014). In this way, nurses and patients are sitting in the realm of the profane rather than the sacred.

Nursing has, itself, evolved from an ignominious, sordid and, thus, abject position. Nursing was not an admired profession, and nor was the work safe. In New York in the 1870s, for example, Egenes (2017) reports that when prostitutes were sentenced at court they were given the choice of going to prison or going into hospital service. In the context of pre-Nightingale England, nursing was a profession only pursued by those who would do anything for extra money. It was dangerous, there was no training, no scientific basis to the treatments and no set standards of care. Nursing was then, as it has always been, a 24-hour profession, yet the night (and night-nursing) in the era before electricity, was an unseemly place for women to be (DeLamotte, 1990). As a result, only the particularly desperate nurses accepted night-time work. The enduring image of the slovenly, cynical and uncaring nurse – Sairey Gamp – embodies this past.

Sairey Gamp, a frumpy and callous nurse, is a fictional character brought to life in Charles Dickens' *Martin Chuzzlewit* (1853). Nurse Gamp, unlike most women of the time, is not afraid to work at night. She relieves the day nurse, Mrs Prig, in the care of an ailing man, the following exchange occurs by way of patient handover:

> "anythin' to tell afore you goes, my dear?" asked Mrs Gamp setting her bundle down inside the door and looking affectionately at her partner.
>
> "The pickled salmon," Mrs Prig replied, "is quite delicious. I can partick'ler recommend it. ... The drinks is all good." ...
>
> Mrs Gamp thanked her for these hints, and giving her a friendly good night, held the door open until she had disappeared at the other end of the gallery. Having thus performed the hospitable duty of seeing her safely off, she shut it, locked it on the inside, took up her bundle, walked round the screen and entered on her occupation of the sick chamber.
>
> "A little dull, but not so bad as it might be," Mrs Gamp remarked. "I'm glad to see a parapidge, in case of fire, and lots of roofs and chimley-pots to walk upon."
>
> It will be seen from these remarks that Mrs Gamp was looking out of window. When she had exhausted the prospect, she tried the easy-chair, which she indignantly declared was "harder than a brickbadge". Next she pursued her researches among the physic-bottles, glasses, jugs, and tea-cups; and when she had entirely satisfied her curiosity on all these subjects of investigation, she untied her bonnet-strings and strolled up to the bedside to take a look at the patient.

It is clear from this passage that her patient is the final of Sairey Gamp's concerns, after her own wellbeing and entertainment. The patient is described next.

> A young man – dark and not ill-looking – with long black hair, that seemed the blacker for the whiteness of the bed clothes. His eyes were partly open, and he never ceased to roll his head from side to side upon the pillow, keeping his body almost quiet. He did not utter words; but every now and then gave vent to his restless head – oh, weary, weary hour! – went to and fro without a moment's intermission.
>
> Mrs Gamp solaced herself with a pinch of snuff, and stood looking at him with her head inclined a little sideways, as a connoisseur might gaze upon a doubtful work of art. By degrees, a horrible remembrance of one branch of her calling took possession of the woman; and stopping down, she pinned his wandering arms against his sides, to see how he would look if laid out as a dead man. Hideous as it may

appear, her fingers itched to compose his limbs in that last marble attitude.

"Ah!" said Mrs Gamp, walking away from the bed, "he'd make a lovely corpse!"

(pp. 291–292)

Although her charge is clearly distressed and in pain, this nurse, quite remarkable in her callous disregard for his suffering, considers the environment for what comforts it can bring to her. The patient is not only not central in her eyes, but viewed contemptuously. In a final act of dehumanisation, still thinking about herself and likely financial gain, she imagines him after death, and the further money she can make from laying him out. Dickens thus portrays the nurse as simultaneously powerful and loathsome.

According to many literary critics and readers, Charles Dickens is one of the greatest novelists of all time (Gottschall, 2012). His works proved to be lastingly popular, with his stories continuing to be told in various media for over a hundred years, and the characterisations of Victorian life in his novels played a significant influence in raising awareness of, and sympathy for, the plight of the poor and needy in a society that had few social supports and no State-supplied welfare. Dickens unambiguously criticised the brutal system of workhouses, debtor's prisons and orphanages that kept England's poor virtually enslaved (Markel, 2016). Sairey Gamp was one of the most enduring characters he created. She was a nurse who was self-focused and manipulative, generally drunk and the embodiment of a sloppy, self-indulgent caretaker. Untrained, her incompetence is seen as largely stemming from her personal flaws, her intemperance and greed. Her character effectively represented a corrupt, dysfunctional and pathetically inadequate health care system that vulnerable populations were forced to rely upon. Public sympathies for this dire situation eventually led to reforms in government systems, and politicised people like Florence Nightingale to become activists for change. Her lamp, quite literally, took nursing out of the darkness. The public today may no longer recognise the image of nursing projected by Dickens in *Martin Chuzzlewit,* but nursing's roots were here, and perhaps when there are reports of patients fearing a visitation from a nurse, they are unconsciously recalling this vivid image from an abject past.

Struggling to manage the abject

The strict orders about caring and cleanliness promulgated by nursing schools can be read as an attempt to ward off the human impulses to avoid the rigours and horrors of illness. An important decree from Nightingale's time was that nurses were to be "in the world, but not a part of it" (Reverby, 1987, p. 90). This introduces an important and irresolvable paradox for nursing that

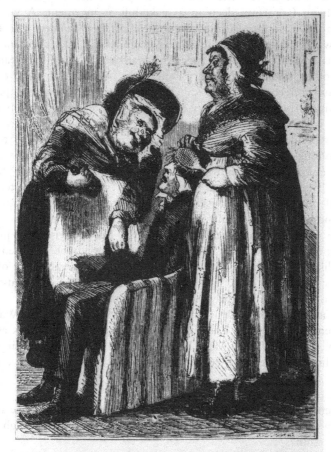

SAIREY GAMP AND BETSEY PRIG PREPARE THEIR PATIENT FOR A JOURNEY.

Figure 4.1 Charles Dickens' fictional nurse, Sairey Gamp, embodies nursing's abject past.

continues today. Nurses, as human beings, have no choice but to be *in* the world and to display ordinary human weaknesses and fears, yet their work requires that they sometimes move beyond that normally expected in society and "descend" into the world of the abject.

This impossible challenge, and the toll it takes on nurses, is evident in a scene from a film created in the period between the First and Second World Wars, *War Nurse* (1930). Hazel Meadows, a naïve young woman, decides to enlist as a nurse in the First World War because she thinks it will be a good place to meet men. She is given a rude awakening when she is summoned to assist the physician on duty and is – in effect –

bombarded with abject encounters. The pair enter a ward filled with patients, lying four rows deep in a makeshift arrangement. A whimpering man with his head bandaged is the centre of their concern. As the new nurse unwraps his bandages, the doctor examines his face, pronouncing that shrapnel is embedded in both eyes. The ward erupts with the heartrending cries of other soldiers who mirror his pain. When one man cries out, another nurse recognises shell shock and calls every available person to restrain him. After this chaotic scene, the exhausted and frightened Nurse Meadows is shown crying herself to sleep. She is soon, however, awoken, as more wounded are incoming. When she protests that she is too tired, the supervising Sister responds, "A nurse is never too tired, nor too sick, nor too cold, nor too hungry. Do you understand?" Nurse Meadows answers, "But I can't look at any more hurt men!". The Sister replies, firmly but not without kindness, "You'll learn to look at men without arms or legs and without faces and you'll smile because they need you". When the nurse expresses shame at her despair, the Sister advises the process of enculturation all nurses undergo, "There's nothing to be ashamed of. We were all like you at first". This excerpt highlights a universal rite of passage for nurses; how they learn to suppress natural reactions of disgust, nausea and fear in order to effectively care for individuals in need.

The tension involved in this suppression is vividly recorded in Walt Whitman's poem "The Wound Dresser" (1897), which recalls his work as a nurse during the American Civil War. In this poem the narrator, dressing terrible wounds, hopes for death to come quickly to his charges who have no hope of cure:

> The crush'd head I dress, (poor crazed hand tear not the bandage away,)
> The neck of the cavalry-man with the bullet through and through
>   I examine,
> Hard the breathing rattles, quite glazed already the eye, yet life struggles
>   hard,
> (Come sweet death! be persuaded O beautiful death!
> In mercy come quickly.)

The wounds the nurse must deal with are described graphically:

> From the stump of the arm, the amputated hand,
> I undo the clotted lint, remove the slough, wash off the matter and
>   blood,
> Back on his pillow the soldier bends with curv'd neck and side falling
>   head,
> His eyes are closed, his face is pale, he dares not look on the bloody stump,
> And has not yet look'd on it.

The nurse continues to provide these clean dressings, despite the presence of gangrenous decay:

> I dress a wound in the side, deep, deep,
> But a day or two more, for see the frame all wasted and sinking,
> And the yellow-blue countenance see./
> I dress the perforated shoulder, the foot with the bullet-wound,
> Cleanse the one with a gnawing and putrid gangrene, so sickening,
>   so offensive,
> While the attendant stands behind aside me holding the tray and pail./
> I am faithful, I do not give out,
> The fractur'd thigh, the knee, the wound in the abdomen,
> These and more I dress with impassive hand, (yet deep in my breast
>   a fire, a burning flame).
>
> (Levine et al., 2016)

The high emotion felt is repressed, the repulsive wounds are tolerated and tended. The narrator articulates this in terms of staying firm ("faithful") to the task, and not giving way, but the conflict between the "impassive hand" and the "burning flame" of indignity and disgust pains the narrator. This poem powerfully shows how, despite their natural impulse to turn away, nurses must instead find ways to internalise repulsion and fear, to serve their patient.

Understanding the abject

Although a large part of contemporary nursing work is situated in this turbulent and traumatic realm (Evans, 2010), maintaining a detached and uncritical attitude means that the abject and profane aspects of nursing remain unaddressed. As a result, many in society – including nurses, nursing scholars, educators and nursing students, alongside the general public – have a limited lexicon with which to describe this work, and its effects on nurses and those in their care. This leads members of all these groups to tend to promulgate existing stereotypes, such as the notion of nurses working only in the realm of the sacred, which makes them angelic and their work "clean". Such unrealistic representations sanitise the realities of nursing and erase many of the complexities involved in professional practice. Failing to recognise darker, more disturbing narratives about nurses and nursing experience – those that subvert the domestic and the sacred – also means that these remain untheorised (McAllister and Brien, 2016).

Bradbury-Jones and Taylor (2014) explain that there are three elements that can assist with understanding how the abject is experienced by both nurses and patients. There is the clean and proper (non-abject) self; there is physical matter which is abject in itself, like blood, vomit and decay; and there are the reactions to encounters with these abject aspects. Kristeva (1982, p.1) points out that the abject additionally "beseeches, worries, and fascinates desire". The abject is thus both disgusting and irresistible, and simultaneously both repulses and summons. It is even more complex, as writing about nursing generally, Evans (2010, p. 199) refers to the nature of nursing as "strange yet compelling" due to the vagaries of abjection: what one nurse may find disgusting and repulsive, another may find challenging and rewarding.

Death and dying

For many people in society, death and dying are at the apex of unmentionable subjects. So much so that, although "end-of-life issues" are beginning to be discussed in a range of public forums from personal memoirs (Berman, 2012) to "Death cafés" (Miles and Corr, 2017), they are still largely taboo. Mary Douglas (2002, p. xi) famously describes a taboo as that which is perceived as "dirty and dangerous", with fear of pollution and contagion prominent in the development and maintenance of such "off limits" topics. It makes sense that palliative care is also considered a contentious space in professional terms because many nurses themselves feel anxious about dealing with death and dying. Many nurses are not ready, or willing, to care for these patients, or feel able to cope with the potentially unpleasant associated tasks (Gillan, van der Riet and Jeong, 2014). There are, however, others who find the work appealing (Oliviere and Hargreaves, 2017).

The notion that the abject can be simultaneously taboo and yet captivating in the context of palliative care nursing is evoked in the films *Magnolia* (Anderson, 1999) and *Chronic* (Franco, 2015). *Magnolia* is a non-linear narrative. The action takes place over one day, during which the stories of a number of characters are cleverly interwoven. One of these stories is that of retired television quiz show producer, Earl Partridge (played by Jason Robards), who is in the late stages of dying from cancer. He is cared for in his home by nurse, Phil Parma (played by Philip Seymour Hoffman). Although *Magnolia* deploys unconventional filmic devices – all the characters, for instance, join in singing a final song at the end of the movie – Nurse Parma plays quite a conventional nurse in the story. He is calm, gentle, competent and respectful. Alongside his expected duties, however, Partridge tasks him with finding his son, Frank, from whom he is estranged, so they can be reconciled before he dies. Although this clearly lays outside the purely medical side of his role, Parma takes his role seriously, showing a kind and selfless humanity. He takes on an extra shift, talks to a number of people about his quest and even awkwardly orders home delivery of a series of pornographic magazines to assist his patient. A profoundly moving scene in the film occurs where Frank (played by Tom Cruise) comes to see his father. As Earl lies mostly quietly, literally on his deathbed, Frank confronts him with how badly he treated his mother – then Earl's wife – when she was dying of cancer.

Parma is shown in the background, clearly uncomfortable, but witnessing the scene and unwilling to desert the patient in his care. As Frank breaks down and sobs, Parma is shown with his head in his hands, but still he remains. Parma's role in this scene is made more poignant by being shown, for the most part, in the background and out of focus. He is thus placed in the same proximity to the scene being played out as the viewer, and it is easy to project the viewer's discomfort onto the nurse.

Writer and director, Paul Thomas Anderson, stated that he wanted to air a number of everyday topics that were not usually featured in film; as he described, "the things that I know as big and emotional are these real intimate everyday moments" (quoted in Patterson, 2000). He describes Parma as a "simple, uncomplicated, caring character" (quoted in Patterson, 2000), as an individual who "really takes pride in the fact that every day he's dealing with life and death circumstances" (quoted in New Line Cinema, 1999). Despite this, Parma also seems a somewhat subdued and lonely character, his life clearly lived through his work, but about which he does not seem to have anyone with which to share any misgivings or grief. Perhaps this characterisation signals a truth about nursing, which is that working with, and in, the abject can be a lonely, isolating experience, one in which few understand the calling and its challenges and rewards.

This aspect of nursing is foregrounded in *Chronic* (2015), a film in which the narrative turns around the life and work of home-based palliative care nurse, David (played by Tim Roth). Written and directed by Michel Franco, the film chronicles a few months in David's life and those of the patients for whom he cares. The film is highly unusual in terms of both this subject matter, and the languid, detailed scenes of David implementing intimate body care. Viewers see him bathing, dressing and feeding dying patients, sensitively interrupting family interactions to dispense medications, or simply joining his patients in reading or some other everyday activity. One of his patients, Sarah, is frail, in pain, her body marred by skin lesions and weakened from an unidentified wasting disease. David is her home-based nurse. He bathes her thoroughly, but gently, not shying away from his client's nudity, skeletal frame and helplessness. It is a scene of extreme, and disturbing, intimacy. Some days later, he is shown washing and prepares Sarah's now-deceased body. He bathes her as tenderly and respectfully as he did when she was alive, but his face is impassive and his feelings are inscrutable. Later that evening, in a conversation with some strangers in a bar, David tells them, perhaps to explain his solo drinking, that his wife, who he calls Sarah, has recently died and that he cared for her. It is unclear, as his patient Sarah was not his wife, whether the lie is simply his way of garnering sympathy for a loss that he might keenly feel or whether he is intentionally being deceptive in order to make himself appear more interesting or worthy of sympathy.

This provides a clue to the film's theme, which may be: Who cares for the caregiver? Another hypothesis as to the film's theme is more nefarious. At one level, he seems caring and attentive but, on another, his motivations and intentions are enigmatic, and even worrisome. Several patients die under David's care. This is unsurprising as they are terminally ill, but incongruities begin to recur which raise doubt as to whether their deaths are natural or assisted. Although *Chronic* is ultimately ambiguous about whether David is an angel of mercy or of death (Davis, 1992), it deals with the euthanasia debate in a subtle, yet insistent, manner. While completely compelling, David's character and motivations are deeply mysterious and uncertain, mirroring deep-seated cultural anxieties about both medically assisted processes of dying and death itself.

This, and the other treatment David provides, also illuminates a number of largely unspoken aspects of dying, and the palliative care nurses offer to those in these final stages of life. David's next patient is an elderly man, John, afflicted by a stroke incurred a number of years before. Whereas Sarah was represented as quite passive, John is angry due to his disability and dependence on his family. David works with him by stretching his stiffened body and setting him small tasks in order that he can engage in at least some measure of self-care and independence. On one occasion, distressed with breathlessness, John clings to David, and David holds him closely, easing his anxiety. Family members watch this embrace and then lodge a complaint about David's behaviour – regarding his intentions as manipulative and possibly sexual. David is prohibited from any further contact with his patient and complies, although reluctantly. The family are seemingly fearful of the intimacy that their father has granted to his nurse. Here the film takes a poignant turn by raising what may be an uncomfortable truth for some families dealing with the impending death of a family member – in hospice-based care, patients often make intimate connections to nurses that can leave family members feeling left out, jealous or outraged (Dowling, 2006). The last patient David cares for in the film, Greg, is a young, physically disabled man, whose mother is taking some respite leave from his care. The two are shown sitting in silence across a table in a park. When David eventually asks Greg if he needs anything, the patient swears at him. This reveals another uncomfortable truth, that chronic and other illnesses make some patients remote, difficult and even unlikeable.

The film is remarkable for its close and determined examination of aspects about end-of-life nursing and death that are not normally depicted in popular culture (McAllister and Brien, 2017). The intimate body care of a dependant and vulnerable patient is rarely pictured and, even rarer, is that the nurse in such proximity to a patient is portrayed as male. Other issues that the film raises that are uncomfortable yet real for contemporary palliative care clinicians are that dying people do request nurses for assistance to die (Street and Kissane, 2001, p. 167). This may be confronting and uncomfortable, but nurses must face the probability that such questions will be asked of them. Another unsettling reality depicted is that nurses frequently work in isolation in home-based palliative care. This places a huge responsibility on them to manage not only a client's physical needs, but the psychological and spiritual struggles that they and family members may be grappling with; issues like loss of control, pain and fear of death (Boston, Bruce and Schreiber, 2011). Finally, the film alludes to a burden that many nurses experience – that they themselves may struggle with personal issues, and even resort to psychological defence mechanisms such as sublimation and projection, to manage their own personal grief and losses, by focusing on the care of others (Abeni et al., 2014).

These portrayals reflect the tension between the profane (illness, dying and death) and the sacred (engaged, selfless care) which is at the heart of why representing characters, and their relationships, in an end-of-life setting, can provide such fruitful subject matter for storytelling (see Brien and Piatti-Farnell, 2016). But, more than this, all three of these nurses also reveal a social paradox. This is that although, as humans, we are frequently disgusted by the physical and mental ravages of disease and death (Curtis, 2007), there are some people who are drawn to the dead and the dying, and society needs this latter group. Professions in this second category would include specialist nurses and doctors, coroners and undertakers. Although the specific tasks undertaken by these professionals in relation to death and dying are only rarely discussed in popular culture, learning about their work is obviously fascinating for audiences, as can be seen in the popularity of a significant number of memoirs of funeral home directors and morticians (Brien, 2017) and others who deal with death in their everyday work, such as those involved in capital punishment (Carter, 2016; Dernley, 2009). This reveals a fascination with the details of death and dying, but when experienced at a "safe" remove (Brien, 2016, 2019). Fictional stories such as *Magnolia* and *Chronic* reveal the ongoing dilemmas that have not been processed by either society in general, or health professionals in particular, about death and dying. They show that simply having a medical discourse to draw upon is not sufficient.

Unimagined horrors

Experiences that incite abjection are those that disturb identity and order, and do not respect rules or borders. In 2005, a climate event occurred in the United States that led to disastrous and unimagined consequences, and in which nurses and doctors were forced to take actions that led to patients' deaths.

Early in the morning of 29 August 2005, a category 5 storm, Hurricane Katrina, made landfall on the gulf coast of the USA causing massive destruction. Cyclonic winds whipped across the country, devastating towns in Mississippi, Florida and Louisiana. Over one thousand people died in the hurricane and subsequent flooding (Knabb, Rhome and Brown, 2005), making it the deadliest United States hurricane to that date. In New Orleans, power lines were brought down and the temperatures inside homes soared above 40 degrees celsius; the Mississippi river burst through levees and unprecedented widespread flooding thwarted evacuations and rescue attempts. For several days, people were stranded on rooftops and in sports stadiums, without adequate food, water, shelter, policing or health care. Hospitals too, often considered indestructible and self-sufficient, were severely affected. Struggling to cope with limited resources after the storm, these hospitals then received large numbers of nursing home residents as well as other injured and ill individuals.

In the documentary *I was there: Hurricane Katrina* (The History Channel, 2015), Henrietta Walton, Nursing Supervisor of the ICU at Charity Hospital in 2005, recalls the experience of working to keep people alive before help came. With floodwaters rising, streets were turned into rivers and the hospital was completely cut off. The inundation destroyed the hospital generators leaving the twelve storey facility totally without power.

> We had to go old school. We had to take out old equipment and use that (for example, self-inflating bags to ventilate patients instead of respirators). Everyone was very mindful that we had to meet basic needs – making sure they [the patients] were clean, given water, keeping them fed as best as possible, and to survive. It was getting kind of hairy because most of the nurses had been working around the clock, no breaks, so it was at that point that we had to kick it in to survival mode.
>
> (4:47/13:47)

As medical journalist Sheri Fink (2009) reported, there was no running water and the sewage system backed up. There was no air conditioning, no functioning elevators and all of the electronic medical equipment such as ventilators, infusion pumps and dialysis machines were useless (Okie, 2008). As patients began to suffer and die due to these conditions, and realising that their evacuation could still be days away, the medical staff gathered to formulate a plan. Patients were organised into three groups and moved to the lower floors, to facilitate the most efficient rescue when it did come. The priority patients to be evacuated would be the "walking wounded", next would be those who needed more assistance, while the third group, and last to leave, would be those under Do Not Resuscitate (DNR) orders.

Exhausted nurses had only comfort measures to offer patients, and a priority for the staff was moving patients safely to the lower floors. This was extremely distressing – carrying or pushing patients down many flights of stairs, administering treatments such as manual or battery-operated suctioning, completing wound care and servicing hygiene needs without running water, offering meagre rations of food and, and in some cases, manually ventilating non-breathing patients. Meanwhile, corpses were decomposing, food was running short, and nurses and doctors began to wonder if they would ever be rescued. When journalists were finally able to inspect the disaster site, Fink released a shocking report:

The smell of death was overpowering the moment a relief worker cracked open one of the hospital chapel's wooden doors. Inside, more than a dozen bodies lay motionless on low cots and on the ground, shrouded in white sheets. Here, a wisp of gray hair peeked out. There, a knee was flung akimbo. A pallid hand reached across a blue gown.

As time went on, some patients became too sick or dependent to move from their beds and so remained in the upper floors where some nurses and doctors attempted to provide them with care (Deichmann, 2007). Some patients died while awaiting evacuation, while others were euthanised. Thus, nurses and doctors were involved in an illegal act of mercy killing that still today remains too controversial to be widely discussed (Okie, 2008).

After five days, the patients and staff were finally evacuated, but according to Okie (2008), by that time, at least thirty-four patients had died, some as a result of medical assistance. It is hard to believe that such a situation could emerge in a modern health care system today. Yet the nurses and doctors were forced into an experience of abject system failure, where some believed it was more humane to kill patients, than to let them await a rescue that may have never come. In studies undertaken on the mental health of nurses following this disaster, it has been reported that up to twenty percent developed symptoms of Post-Traumatic Stress Disorder, although not a single nurse was offered access to the stress management support they had a right to receive (Battles, 2007).

Conclusion

This chapter has discussed a range of circumstances that can be described as abject. Numerous situations have been considered in which nurses in popular culture were challenged to work in a fully engaged and embodied way with patients and communities, while encountering serious obstacles such as tension, conflict, tragedy and pain. These representations have looked beyond the dominant trope of the good and trustworthy nurse working in a rational, functioning health care system, to explore darker, more subversive dimensions of nursing, to shed light on aspects of society and nursing culture that are problematic, but so common as to have become normalised and, therefore, often almost invisible. Ideally, nurses are prepared for experiences of pain and suffering, but it may not be humanly possible to fully prepare for traumatic and horrifying events. To deal with the abject, many nurses learn to use protective coping strategies to distance themselves from revulsion and fear. They may also use peer support, gallows humour and rationalisation to relieve intense feelings and provide some catharsis. It is important, however, that nurses not just endure, but process, abject encounters in order that learning can result and the situation does not become a haunting, unending trauma.

In *Chronic*, the RN David, and in *Magnolia*, the RN Phil, work with the abject body – handling cachectic dying bodies with grace and self-effacement, and bearing witness to realistically portrayed final days that are not the peaceful, easy and acquiescent "good deaths" that proliferate in public imagination. Both nurses complete this work, not in a perfunctory manner, or neglectfully as Sairey Gamp, but with mindful tenderness and respect. While family members and even sometimes the patients themselves are repulsed by the gruesome processes involved in dying, these nurses appear stoic and unaffected. Trudy Rudge and Dave Holmes suggest that nurses are supposed to act in this way – to sublimate any personal negative feelings and present a convincing façade and, in doing so, assuage the cycle of disgust (2009). However, it is also made clear in both *Magnolia* and *Chronic*, as well as in the reporting about, and retellings of, the aftermath of Hurricane Katrina, that the emotional toll of nursing is as much, or more, of a burden for the nurse to bear, as the physical work. In this way, popular culture is able to illuminate a subversive truth about nursing work that is otherwise difficult to articulate and describe.

References

Abeni M, Magni M, Conte M, Mangiacavalli S, Pochintesta L, Vicenzi G, Feretti V, Pompa A, Cocito F, Klersy C and Corso A (2014) Psychological care of caregivers, nurses and physicians: A study of a new approach *Cancer Medicine* 3(1): 101–110.

Allan H, Traynor M, Kelly D and Smith P (2016) *Understanding Sociology in Nursing*. London: Sage.

Anderson P (dir) (1999) *Magnolia*. Film. New York: New Line Cinema.

Battles E (2007) An exploration of post-traumatic stress disorder in emergency nurses following Hurricane Katrina *Journal of Emergency Nursing* 33(4): 314–318.

Berman J (2012) *Dying in Character: Memoirs on the End of Life*. Amherst: University of Massachusetts Press.

Boston P, Bruce A, and Schreiber R (2011) Existential suffering in the palliative care setting: an integrated literature review *Journal of Pain and Symptom Management* 41(3): 604–618.

Bradbury-Jones C, Taylor J, Kroll T and Duncan F (2014) Domestic abuse awareness and recognition among primary healthcare professionals and abused women: A qualitative investigation *Journal of Clinical Nursing* 23(21–2): 3057–3068.

Brien D L (2017) Narratives of death and dying from one remove: Surveying the undertaker's memoir *TEXT: Journal of Writing and Writing Courses* special issue 38. Available at: www.textjournal.com.au/speciss/issue38/Brien.pdf.

Brien D L (2019) Modelling the good death in memoir In Joseph S, Avieson B and Giles F (eds) *Still Here: Memoirs of Trauma and Loss*. London: Routledge, 84–97.

Brien D L and Piatti-Farnell L eds (2016) Writing death and the Gothic *TEXT: Journal of Writing and Writing Courses* special issue 35. Available at: www.textjournal.com.au/speciss/issue35/content.htm.

Carter T (2016) *The Executioner's Redemption: A Story of Violence, Death, and Saving Grace*. St Louis: Concordia Publishing House.

Curtis V (2007) Dirt, disgust and disease: A natural history of hygiene *Journal of Epidemiology and Community Health* 61(8): 660–664.

D L (2016) Making stories of our own ends: Two Australian memoirs of dying *TEXT: Journal of Writing and Writing Courses* special issue 35. Available at: www.textjournal. com.au/speciss/issue35/Brien.pdf.

Davis C (1992) Nurse as angel of mercy *Literature and Medicine* 11(1): 88–89.

DeLamotte E (1990) *Perils of the Night: A Feminist Study of Nineteenth-Century Gothic.* Oxford: Oxford University Press on Demand.

Deichmann R (2007) Code blue: a Katrina physician's memoir. Bloomington: Rooftop Publishing.

Dernley S (2009) *The Hangman's Tale: Memoirs of a Public Executioner.* London: Pan Macmillan.

Dickens C (1853) *Martin Chuzzlewit.* Philadelphia: Getz, Buck & Co.

Douglas M (2002) *Purity and Danger: An Analysis of Concept of Pollution and Taboo.* London: Routledge.

Dowling M (2006) The sociology of intimacy in the nurse-patient relationship *Nursing Inquiry* 20(23): 48–54.

Doyle K, Hungerford C and Cruickshank M (2014) Reviewing tribunal cases and nurse behaviour: Putting empathy back into nurse education with Bloom's taxonomy *Nurse Education Today* 34(7): 1069–1073.

Egenes K (2017) History of nursing In Roux G and Halstead J (eds) *Issues and Trends in Nursing: Essential Knowledge for Today and Tomorrow.* New York: Jones and Bartlett, 1–26.

Evans A (2010) Strange yet compelling: Anxiety and abjection in hospital nursing In Rudge T and Holmes D (eds) *Abjectly Boundless: Boundaries, Bodies and Health Work.* Surrey: Ashgate, 199–211.

Fink, S (2009) The Deadly Choices at Memorial. Propublica. Accessed at: www. propublica.org/article/the-deadly-choices-at-memorial-826.

Fleischer M (1936) *A Song A Day.* Cartoon. New York: Fleischer Productions.

Foth T, Lauzier K and Antweiler K (2017) The limits of a theory of recognition: Toward a nursing ethics of vulnerability In Foth T, Holmes D, Hülsken-Giesler M, Kreutzer S and Remmers H (eds) *Critical Approaches in Nursing Theory and Nursing.* Osnabrück: V&R Unipress, 113–127.

Franco M (dir) (2015) *Chronic.* Film. Los Angeles: Lucia Films.

Gillan P, van der Riet P and Jeong S (2014) End of life care education, past and present: A review of the literature *Nurse Education Today* 34(3): 331–342.

Gottschall J (2012) *The Storytelling Animal: How Stories Make Us Human.* London: Houghton Mifflin Harcourt.

History Channel (2015) *I Was There. Hurricane Katrina: Heroes of Charity Hospital.* Available at: www.history.com/topics/natural-disasters-and-environment/i-was-there-hur ricane-katrina-heroes-of-charity-hospital-video.

Holmes D, Perron A and O'Byrne P (2006) Understanding disgust in nursing: Abjection, self and the other *Research and Theory for Nursing Practice: An International Journal* 20(4): 305–315.

Knabb R, Rhome J and Brown D (December 20, 2005) National Hurricane Center. *Hurricane Katrina: August 23–30, 2005.* Tropical Cyclone Report). Miami: United States National Oceanic and Atmospheric Administration's National Weather Service.

Kristeva J (1982) Approaching abjection *Oxford Literary Review* 5: 125–149.

Lee B (1998–2009) *All Saints.* Television series. Australia: Seven Network.

Levine R, Elliott M, Gustafson S, Hungerford A and Loeffelholz M. (eds.) (2016). *The Norton Anthology of American Literature,* vol. B. New York: Norton, 2279–2281.

Markel H (2016) Was Charles Dickens the first celebrity medical spokesman *PBS News Hour*. Available at: www.pbs.org/newshour/health/was-charles-dickens-the-first-celebrity-medical-spokesman.

McAllister M and Brien D L (2016) Narratives of the "not-so-good nurse": Rewriting nursing's virtue script *Hecate* 41(1 and 2): 79–97.

McAllister M and Brien D L (2017) Death, nursing and writing ambiguous characters *TEXT: Journal of Writing and Writing Courses* special issue 45. Available at: www.text journal.com.au/speciss/issue45/content.htm.

Miles L and Corr C (2017) Death cafe: What is it and what we can learn from it *OMEGA-Journal of Death and Dying* 75(2): 151–165.

New Line Cinema. (1999) Magnolia Production Notes *Cinemareview.com*. Available at: www.cinemareview.com/production.asp?prodid=813.

Okie S (2008) Dr. Pou and the Hurricane — Implications for Patient Care during Disasters *New England Journal of Medicine* 358(1): 1–5.

Oliviere D and Hargreaves R (2017) *Good Practices In Palliative Care: A Psychosocial Perspective*. New York: Routledge.

Patterson J (2000) Magnolia maniac *The Guardian*. 10 March. Available at: www.the guardian.com/film/2000/mar/10/culture.features.

Reverby S (1987) *Ordered to Care: The Dilemma of American Nursing, 1850–1945*. Cambridge, MA: Cambridge University Press.

Roden C (1998) Yesterday's news. *All Saints* episode 21, season 1. Television series. Sydney: Twilight Productions.

Rudge T and Holmes D eds (2009) *Abjectly Boundless: Boundaries, Bodies and Health Work*. Surrey: Ashgate.

Selwyn E (dir) (1930) *The War Nurse*. Film. Hollywood: MGM.

Street A and Kissane D (2001) Discourses of the body in euthanasia: Symptomatic, dependent, shameful and temporal *Nursing Inquiry* 8(3): 162–172.

Whitman W (2016) The wound dresser In Levine R, Elliott M, Gustafson S, Hungerford A and Loeffelholz M (eds). *The Norton Anthology of American Literature*, Volume B. New York: Norton, 2279–2281.

5 Apparitions, lost souls and healing spaces

Introduction

In the fifth episode of the third season of *Nurse Jackie* (2011), Hospital Administrator Gloria Akilitis (played by Anna Deavere Smith) approaches Jackie and conspiratorially asks her, "Have you ever stolen anything?". Nurse Jackie responds impassively, but honestly, "Yes, many times". Akilitis surprisingly answers, "Good! Chapel. Half hour". So begins a seemingly light and humorous scenario that, when unpacked, reveals the ambivalence in which society holds once sacred, healing spaces such as hospitals, and the significance this has for health services and those who work within them. The story continues as the nurses enter the small chapel, which is a familiar room for the staff who use it as a space in which to take breaks, rest, gossip or give each other support. Removed from the harsh lights and loud noises of the busy hospital, the chapel is a peaceful, reflective space. Ornately carved entrance doors and subdued wall lamps make the room feel welcoming. Light filtering through the colourful stained-glass windows illuminate the reverent faces of the statues of Jesus, Mary and Saints standing in the shadows, plus something jarring in this environment, Akilitis pushing a furniture trolley. When Jackie asks dryly, "What's with the hardware?", Akilitis growls, "The diocese is deconsecrating this chapel!" When Jackie asks what that means, Akalitis exclaims, "They're taking my statues!" Standing in front of a statue of the Virgin Mary, Akalitis continues,

> Of all the statues in here, this is the one that matters to me. She's tall, she's got a lot on her mind, and I relate. Also, she's not judgmental. That's something I'm working on. It's irrational, but that's the nature of faith.

Pausing, she looks at the nurses, and then explains, "We're stealing her. Sorry to make you an accessory". When Jackie acquiesces, Akalitis adds, warningly: "You were never here! But since you are, strap Mary to the dolly and follow me!" This scene echoes a sentiment expressed by Reimer-Kirkham et al. (2012) in which they argue that, in recent years, there has been a shift in attitude towards the role of the sacred in health care. Alongside the drive towards holistic and person-centred care, there has been a resurgence of religious and spiritual plurality in health care.

Once steeped in religious iconography and ritual, the sacred healing spaces that characterised hospital design have been largely replaced. In the process, contemporary, modernist and functional architecture almost eclipses vestiges of an important religious past in hospitals. But looking closely at older campuses such as St Bartholomew's Hospital in London, or the Hôtel Dieu in Paris, centuries old gateways, windows, gargoyles, crucifixes, apses, foyers, graveyards and shrines remain as reminders of a more spiritual past. For centuries, hospitals and healing were associated with religious orders. Every religion articulates a mission to care for the sick, believing that in tending to the physical body there is opportunity to also nurture the soul (Grundmann, 1990). For this reason, there is a deep connection between the body and the spirit within health care. Religious orders of monks and nuns also played an important role in the history of nursing (Donahue, 2011). Indeed, up until the late twentieth century, in many parts of the world, registered nurses were, like nuns, referred to as "Sister". Nursing was considered a calling and lifetime vocation, where the privilege of caring was of greater significance than wages, status or working conditions. More recently, however, changing social movements – the rise of secularism, science and managerialism – have seen religion and spirituality virtually disappear from health care. However, even amongst nurses and doctors committed to evidence-based practice and bio-medical advances, this loss is deeply felt.

In the earlier chapters of this volume, numerous examples of representations of nurses working within the realm of the profane have emphasised the ways the image in which the "good" nurse and nursing work as sacred can be transgressed. This chapter focuses on the ways nurses relate to sacred and spiritual aspects of nursing that may appear to belong in nursing's past – and which seem to transgress the scientific ethos of modern health care – but which may still be influencing thoughts, values, practices and nursing identity today.

Rituals to create healing spaces

Nursing has long been engaged in various rituals to promote patient well-being. These rituals may have been based on tradition, or spiritual/religious reasons, or come about because of their therapeutic value. Post-mortem care, also known as "the Last Offices", is a nursing practice that is taken very seriously, and usually conducted in pairs. The opening and closing of windows at set times, the removal of flower vases at night, ensuring specific space is maintained between beds, daily baths and daily linen changes are just some of the practices that persist today, some due to – but some without – reasons based in evidence. These rituals offer deep insight into the meaning, purpose and value of nursing in society.

Sandy Bayley (2015) recalls ritual actions she was ordered to perform in a medical ward in Adelaide, Australia, many years ago:

Loman Ward had two long rows of beds, one each side of the ward. We were not permitted to go off duty until all the beds in the ward had their counterpanes hanging at exactly the same length each side. All the bed wheels had to run in line with the floorboards and the Holland blinds at the windows had to be lowered to equal length all along the windows. Sister OCD used a measuring tape to check. Pillow case openings had to face away from the door; however, with a door at each end of the ward, I faced the dilemma of which door did they mean. The origin of this rule was a practical one, derived from the days when hospitals were in tents. Keeping the open end of the pillowcase away from the tent flap reduced the amount of dirt that ended up inside the pillowcase.

(eBook, Chapter 12, p. 4)

There are still nurses today who maintain such habits, perhaps because it helps to make the ward look orderly, or perhaps just because this is what they were taught.

Other rituals assist in helping people cope with the reality that health care is not always about keeping people alive. Indeed, in some contexts of care, death is almost a daily expectation. In many residential care settings, rituals are enacted upon the death of a resident – in one instance, the consoling poem "The Little Ship" (often also read at funerals) is posted on a deceased resident's door and remains there until after the person's funeral; in another, a white rose is placed on the bed of the resident who has died; in yet another, staff attend the funeral and form an honour guard (Bern-Klug, 2011). These rituals restore a sense of meaning and connection and are reminders that while it is normal to die in advanced old age, the death of one member of a community is a loss for everyone in that community.

Haunting places and apparitions

During the Industrialisation period, hospitals began to be built on a huge scale. Their sheer size, and ability to accommodate thousands of patients at one time, has stimulated the imagination of storytellers for generations. Psychiatric asylums, in particular, have often been featured in horror stories and films. The eerie feelings associated with such structures are evoked in this excerpt from the memoir of a mental health nurse who worked at Danvers State Asylum in Massachusetts, USA, in the late 1940s.

Even back then its time worn buildings held a long history. Danvers had been a state institution for the insane for many, many years. It had acquired an aura of mystique that had become a source of local fascination. The facility was completely isolated from the surrounding communities, sitting high on a hill surrounded by a large tract of wooded land. The trees obscured its physical presence. It lay hidden like some long ignored malignancy. The main drive leading up to Danvers was a winding narrow road gradually ascending to the main gates. The entrance brought to mind visions of the entrance to Dante's inferno. My first impression of the facility was one of awe. ... At the top, Danvers stood like some gothic castle, a forbidding structure that served as a solid reminder of how much people had always feared and shunned madness. Thick stone walls guarded the melancholy secrets of that place. Despite its seclusion, everyone in the area knew of the insane asylum high up on the hill. It was a place shrouded in modern day myth and legend, a place that in time would leave its indelible mark on me. ... Masses of creeping vines wound their way up the stone walls that had taken on a dull gray tint. The sprawling complex ... included a cemetery and a farm nestled besides its forty buildings. It was its own closed community. ... its weathered but pristine appearance hiding the squalor and human sadness that lay inside. When I looked at it for the first time, I felt the visceral fear I believe all of us have when confronting something so far removed from what we consider normal.

(Stillwell, 2004, pp. 1–2)

The excerpt makes clear that nurses were not immune from feelings of fear and trepidation approaching such hospitals. But not only do people find such buildings frightening, they continue to hold negative views about the nurses who work in their modern equivalent – mental health services. Gouthro (2009) argues that this is because representations of asylum care – depicted in many stories about mental illness even today – involved the management of large numbers of patients with few resources. Asylum care was by its nature restrictive, ritualised, rigid and controlling. Nurses who worked in them have been similarly construed.

The following scene from *The Snake Pit* (Litvak, 1948) reinforces the image. Virginia Cunningham, a young woman who has had a breakdown following significant trauma, has experienced a deterioration in her mental state and, as a result, has been transferred to a secure ward, where unsettled and floridly psychotic patients are being kept. Her doctor is escorted through the maze of locked doors, by a silent, stern, efficient nurse, holding a large set of keys. A noisy, chaotic scene unfolds where between screams and ecstatic singing, patient after patient accosts the doctor, begging for attention. The nurse pushes each of them away, making a pathway through which the doctor can safely pass. Finally, the nurse unlocks the fourth door and stands aside. The doctor approaches a solitary woman who barefoot and bound by a straitjacket, stands by a barred window. She turns to the doctor and says "Hello Doctor Kip. Sorry Doctor, I guess I wasn't up to one. I tried, I really did, but I just couldn't make it". The doctor reassures Virginia that it wasn't her fault and asks if the restraints can be removed. The nurse protests, "But doctor, the instructions we got from ...", but the doctor interrupts, saying, "Never mind that, take them off". Virginia is released from the physical restraints but enters a room of disturbed patients pacing the room. The doctors have departed, leaving very few nurses to manage the chaos. There are patients clanging imaginary bells, cackling with laughter, one praying on the floor, another reciting a forceful speech, another taking patients' temperatures with an imaginary thermometer. Virginia asks who this woman is, and when told that she is Miss Somerville, realises that she used to be the nurse in charge of one of the wards.

In this important film exposing shocking standards of care for patients, Litvak (1948) has also made an insightful comment that being immersed in such an unholy place can have devastating effects on the health and wellbeing of the nurses who work there. Thankfully, mental health nurses no longer work in these contexts or conditions, yet the stereotypes about them persist and it is important that new narratives of contemporary mental health care be created and promulgated so that attitudes about this kind of nursing changes (Cleary et al., 2018).

Night terrors

Even though nurses are trained in, and endorse, evidence-based practice, they are not above believing in superstitions. One such belief is that the full moon exacerbates physical and mental disturbances, so much so that this has been termed "The Transylvanian", or "Lunar", effect (Owens and McGowan, 2006). Many mental health nurses, for instance, believe that patients with schizophrenia deteriorate during the time of the full moon (Barr, 2000). A significant number of Emergency Department staff insist that violence increases substantially during the full moon (Snelson, 2004), and there have been studies that indicate an increase in the number of births at this time (Bosanquet, 2001) – which explains why many midwives dread the night shift on a full moon – although there are other studies that dispute these findings (Margot, 2015). Despite science not supporting the phenomenon, many nurses continue to hold firmly to its existence (Foster and Roenneberg, 2008). Christie Watson (2019) is one nurse who insists on its veracity, writing in her memoir:

> There is no scientific evidence that more babies are born during full moons, but I've lived with three midwives: science must be wrong. The morning after a full-moon shift they are always late, stressed and more tired: "Haven't sat down all night! Completely full, and backed up. It's no wonder we all try and roster ourselves on crescent-moon weekends".
>
> (p. 90)

This is one example of how nurses work in liminal spaces – existing between, and crossing, the borders between reason and unreason (or between science and conviction), between day and night, and life and death (McAllister, 2017). These contexts in which nurses work are simultaneously familiar and strange. They are familiar because nurses regularly participate in such challenging human ordeals, and strange because the meaning of these experiences are rarely discussed or commented upon in scholarship, and thus the profession has not yet developed a collective understanding of them. One familiar, yet strange, experience, is the night shift. The night shift takes place when most people are asleep, and, especially for new nurses, can be frightening and unpredictable. A ghostly quiet descends on hospitals in the later evening when the hustle and bustle of routines have ceased. The evening meal has been served and cleared away, most staff and visitors have departed, the lights are subdued and, whenever possible, patients are left to try to gain the benefits of a restful sleep. But the illness processes do not abate and neither do the treatments. Nurses – often in pairs but sometimes alone – must monitor patients' vital signs and administer therapies quietly and unobtrusively.

There is a large body of research on the impact of night shift and nursing. A recent review of this literature revealed numerous issues that have potential to impact negatively on nurses working rotating night shifts (Tahghighi et al., 2017). Research into the night shift has focused on its health implications for nurses (Books et al., 2017) including in terms of disruption to circadian rhythms and risks of cancer and diabetes (Papantoniou et al., 2018), stress (Lin et al., 2015) and disturbed sleep patterns (Beebe et al., 2017). There are also negative implications for the safety of both patients and nurses (Cho et al., 2016). The literature finds that, although working at night has numerous negative ramifications, producing "physical discomforts such as sleep deprivation for long periods, restriction of family and social life, changes in mood and concentration level, and others which appear as factors causing wear and psychological suffering" (Silveira, 2016, p. 3680), there is a general lack of understanding in terms of workers realising "the implications and meanings of the night journey to their life and work" (Silveira, Camponogara and Beck, 2016, p. 3685), meaning that the night shift is a relatively unexplored space in terms of its social and cultural meanings. A rare exception is Brown and Brooks' (2002) research into nurses' emotional experience of night nursing. As nursing lacks a collective understanding of the night shift, nurses are not well prepared to cope with its special demands and pressures. One way that nurses do aim to cope with the night shift is to support each other through conversation and, sometimes, the sharing of thrilling stories, many of which are about ghostly apparitions and other supernatural occurrences on the wards (McAllister and Brien, 2019).

Unlike the sleeping patients and absent hospital staff, nurses remain on high alert on night shifts, so that they can respond to the unexpected (Benner, Tanner and Chesla, 2009), which is one reason why they, more than other employees, are sensitive to what can be described as *unusual* goings on, particularly at night. According to a study by Brayne, Lovelace and Fenwick (2008), many nurses appreciate that strange phenomenon can be meaningful signals, such as to impending changes in a patient's status, and should not be ignored. Nurses are, thus, highly attuned to hearing, seeing or sensing things that are untoward, but subdued lighting and shadows can play tricks on perception and sounds heard in the quiet of the night can take on unnerving qualities.

Linked to this familiarity with strange phenomena, nurses also very quickly become accustomed to death, dying and suffering. Nurses spend lengthy periods of time with dying patients and their family. There is an expectation that nurses be ready to support the spiritual needs of dying people and their families, although many nurses have not received specialised training or supervision in such skills (Ladd et al., 2013). Nurses who work in areas such as palliative care quickly come to learn that not everyone responds predictably to medical treatments – there can be sudden episodes of deterioration, or lucidity, that baffle experts and cannot be explained by medical science (Agrillo, 2011; Betty, 2006). Nurses are also in the position of witnessing patients' end of life experiences and even report their own (Brayne, Lovelace and Fenwick, 2008; Fenwick and Brayne, 2011).

With all these elements taken into account, it is not surprising that nurses' ghost stories abound. While this practice and the resulting discourse may be dismissed as vernacular, it is also replete with meaning about nursing culture. While many of these stories are published informally on blogs (Redding, 2016; Smith, 2018; Steffck, 2016) and in a small number of popular book-length collections (Betters, 2014; Garcez, 2013), nurses' ghost stories have rarely been discussed in academic literature, and thus little is known about their function and meaning.

When nurses are together in the subdued light of the nurses' station, they love to talk to each other, for the work they do – and the things they witness – are often extreme and necessitate a form of debriefing. These stories may also provide a welcome reprieve from the constancy of technical discourse that preoccupies most health care professionals. This talk and storytelling thus serve an important social and cultural function. Not only does it enable nurses to process a complex unfolding of events (Sandelowski, 1994) and provides relief, it can also facilitate support and validation and a sense of connection and belonging. In this way, the sharing of stories, particularly the dark and strange tales shared on night shift, can build a stronger professional identity.

Nurses' ghost stories

Despite the scientific-technical basis of nurses' training and much medical practice, the telling and re-telling of ghost stories is a long-standing practice within the profession. Although largely shrouded in secrecy, there are certain rules around when they are told – including, for example, that they are mostly told at night, in the nurses' station, and only between nurses. The eerie nature of these tales is worthy of close analysis because this can deepen understanding of cultural anxieties that may otherwise be difficult to speak about, but which nonetheless affect public thought and action (Piatti-Farnell, 2018; Spooner, 2006). For Briggs, the characteristic features of a ghost story – where there is "ambivalence of tension between certainty and doubt, between the familiar and the feared, between rational occurrence and the inexplicable" (2012, p. 176) – are what makes such stories so powerful, and can be posited as a reason for their endurance in both practice and popular culture.

The patrolling ghost of Adelaide Billings is a story often repeated in Brisbane, Australia. It is believed by some that the Adelaide Billings Ward in Brisbane's (now-demolished) Royal Children's Hospital in Brisbane was haunted by the nurse after whom it was named. Greatly loved and admired in her lifetime, Matron Billings was honoured after her death by the naming of a ward after her. Thereafter, she was seen to haunt the ward. According to one story, a male nurse found her busily filling a burette one night. He thought her face was vaguely familiar but did not recognise her at the time and thought no more about it until he glanced at a photograph of Matron Billings hanging in the lobby and realised that he had seen a ghost (Brisbane History, 2010). On other occasions, she was observed touring the ward at night checking on her tiny patients, stroking foreheads, tucking in bedclothes and straightening pillows. As of 2011, some forty staff from the Royal Brisbane and Women's Hospital had reported encountering the former matron's ghost (Gough, 2011). Such ghosts, according to Bennett and Royle (2016, p. 187), involve:

> the idea of a spectre, an apparition of the dead, a revenant, the dead returned to a kind of spectral existence – an entity not alive but also not quite, not finally, dead. Ghosts disturb our sense of the separation of the living from the dead – which is why they can be so frightening, so uncanny … Ghosts are paradoxical since they are both fundamental to the human, fundamentally human, and a denial or disturbance of the human, the very being of the inhuman.

This nursing ghost story is quite typical of others shared by nurses in a number of ways (McAllister and Brien, 2019). First, it does not feature the Gothic trope of the witch or ugly crone so familiar in other ghost stories. The crone figure reveals an anxiety about the loss of youth and the decay of old age (Horner and Zlosnik, 2016). Rather, Adelaide Billings is a maternal and helpful ghost who is old, wise and comforting. Importantly, she is a ghost who comes to nurses at night, when they are alone, and helps them to achieve their tasks. Such a story underscores the reality that such women are absent in many nurses' real lives, and thus the ghost operates as a manifestation of what Zizek (2009) describes as an absent presence. That is, the ghost's appearance, and provision of safety to those in need, is present in this apparition, but absent in reality. That this ghostly nurse is always present, watching and waiting, suggests that such extraordinary help is needed to make the system function correctly and safely.

Unsettled and unsettling stories

Narratives such as these are unsettling as, in contrast to techno-rational scientific medical discourse that imbues contemporary health care, the events they portray are supernatural and inexplicable. When set in hospitals, fictional ghost stories are more than unsettling – they are particularly frightening because they often draw upon gruesome illnesses and conditions and terrifying medical procedures, and involve confinement in eerie and often haunted spaces. These stories also feature staff who are hypervigilant and controlling (or, conversely, unaware, callous or worse), and whose specialised medical knowledge is mystifying and unnerving. Fear of the dark – or a fear of possible or imagined dangers or dangerous individuals concealed by that darkness – is a common phobia (Marks, 1969), and regularly used in horror films. Horror stories featuring nurses are thus often set in the night time; where the light plays tricks, and where strange noises can prompt wild imaginings.

In Jaume Balaguero's *Fragile* (2005), a horror film set in a dilapidated children's hospital located on an inhospitable and isolated island, the central figure, a nurse (Amy Nicholls, played by Calista Flockhart), is herself a damaged and fragile figure, but she must step up and be her patients' – the children's – protector. During the day, nothing untoward seems to happen but, at night, in the shadowy wards, unexplainable injuries to the children occur; objects are moved when no one is around them; staff go missing; and children see things that the adults do not. As Carter (2009) explains, the experience of illness often provokes feelings of vulnerability. She writes:

> Patients are put in a passive position, where they depend on the technical knowledge and professional skills of the provider, often a previously unfamiliar individual ... [they] depend on providers to help, to be worthy of trust, to respond morally to their suffering and vulnerabilities, and provide ethically sensitive care.
>
> (p. 393)

The anxiety engendered by the vulnerability of becoming a patient is magnified when set in the context of the night time, where the light is dim and the shadows long, the lack of visibility and the unusual quiet amplifying the tension. In both these films, nurses also suffer significant trauma on the night shift. Ghostly figures and apparitions are symbolic manifestations of the trauma experienced by both nurses and patients. As Laredo (2018, p. 70) explains, trauma is the result of an overwhelming experience that compromises one's ability to cope with the emotions that arise from that experience and can lead to a split between the conscious self and the traumatised Other, that does not allow trauma to be accessed by the conscious self. This split creates gaps in memory that frustrate the survivor's ability to construct a coherent narrative of their trauma. Because of this, trauma can return in the form of unconscious repetition. These stories are not about healing, transformation or redemption, but about chaos, and the ghosts in these films are manifestations of that disorder. For Kristeva (1982), the real horror in ghosts is around that which lies within, and what ghosts reveal about the inner turmoil and terror. As Virginia Woolf wrote in her essay on the Supernatural in fiction in 1918, such stories are most disturbing when they "terrify us not by the ghosts of the dead, but by those ghosts which are living within ourselves" (1966, p. 294).

Fears revealed

These stories also reveal that "fear of death" persists within nurses' thoughts as it does in Australian society (Wiese et al., 2015). In many cultures, death is a such a difficult life issue to discuss that it is recognised as a taboo (Bowen, 2018). Although it appears antithetical to their role, nursing as a sub-culture within society also struggles to discuss death openly (Lorenza et al., 2017) and thus caring for people who may die is a daunting task. Nurses' fear of their own deaths is also confronted when they work with patients who may die (Braun, Gordon and Uziely, 2010). Yet, paradoxically, at the same time, unlike the public, nurses cannot easily deny end-of-life experiences, as they occur regularly in their working lives.

Second, nurses on night shift often work on their own, or without adequate supervision (Dawson et al., 2014). As a result, their anxiety is high and they fear what may happen, or has happened, to patients. This fear is normally repressed into the unconscious, thus allowing nurses to turn up for night shift and to work as if it is just another shift. The sharing of ghost stories is an outlet for this repression and may also work as cautionary tales for the uninitiated. The moral of such stories is always, "be aware that danger lurks here" (McAllister and Brien 2019).

Thirdly, and paradoxically, nurses readily believe the supernatural and extra-sensory perceptions in these tales. Thus, despite being trained to be logical and technically precise, they still hold beliefs in the intuitive and the spiritual. This is interesting because nursing theorists talk about "intuitive knowing" and "emotional work" in relation to nursing (Cowling III, Smith and Watson, 2008). This theory points to the limits to logical-rational discourse; how it fails to explain the entirety of health-care work and does not embrace the idea that there is a "form of knowing" that nurses are privy to. This is why many nurses value the idea of "embodied knowing" (Nelson, 2007). This is a form of knowledge that incorporates an intuitive and intimate knowledge of a patient, as well as an acknowledgment of the humble, and open, stance of unknowing. Being unknowing acknowledges that one does not have all the answers to a patient's predicament, and that to truly learn about him or her, the nurse needs to step into their shoes by listening, learning and feeling with the other (Wright and Brajtman, 2011).

Catharsis and understanding

Nurses sometimes work on the periphery of knowing (they know some of what doctors know, but not all, and they may be privy to information that cannot be shared) and being on this edge is precarious and risky. Sometimes, too, the issues that nurses must encounter, often on their own, is beyond their psychological capacity (Beck, 2011). This includes suffering, brutality, death, the abjectness of illness and disease, as well as working within neo-liberal soulless institutions directed by sometimes irrational and contradictory policies. Being unable to deal with the trauma of these issues, as well as the trauma that patients are going through, leads to repression and other ways to cover up the pain. But as Freud (1957) [1915] famously suggested, this repression constantly returns, in the form of nightmares, unrest, vigilance and expectations of further suffering. Yet, despite frightening experiences, isolation and working outside the boundaries of knowledge, nurses are expected by society, their colleagues and from themselves, to cope (Jones and Kelly, 2014).

Engaging with horror narratives permits readers, audiences and other media consumers to connect with the macabre and the horrific at a safe remove without any risk of physical danger (Hughes, 2015), and for the pleasurable frisson this provides (Royle, 2003). As Piatti-Farnell and Brien (2015) suggest, one of the purposes that the Gothic can serve is that of catharsis. Gothic works are reflexive, standing in for what is feared, allowing consumers to virtually confront and experience what engenders anxiety and uncertainty (Spooner, 2006). The lure of the Gothic in these stories is compelling, because the health journey is, at times, terrifying and anxiety inducing for both patients and nurses. In particular, the difficult and sometimes traumatic activities and issues that occur either expectedly, or unexpectedly, in the process of health care, can come back to nurses (and patients) via memories and dreams. Such uncanny occurrences, using Piatti-Farnell's conception (2017), can be seen to "haunt" both nursing itself as well as it's representation in popular culture. Yashinsky (2006) similarly suggests that ghost stories in health are a way to acknowledge spirituality and mystery in the clinical world. When nurses journey into the unknown and the uncanny with their night shift rituals and shared storytelling, they may be unconsciously protesting the marginalisation of spirituality and unique patient experiences in health care. In essence, this behaviour (including storytelling) preserves the importance of spirit and mystery, providing a way for a long-silenced part of health care and nursing to be articulated and heard.

Night shift rituals and shared storytelling may thus be much more than a personal safety valve or moment of frisson-filled pleasure. Understanding such deeper layers of meaning and significance have implications for nursing practice and areas for improvements to health care. For example, in *Fragile*, the supernatural aspects of the story are underpinned by problems associated with short staffing, antiquated and inadequate facilities, and the past abuse of patients. Such a ghost story allows these unspeakable, alternative worlds of nursing to be articulated and (vicariously) experienced. This, in turn, alerts nurses to things that may become taken for granted. As Grice-Swenson (2015) argues, there is need to heed the voice of night nurses who feel insufficiently supported and undervalued. Her study of night nurses found that many do not feel safe or supported on night duty, even though they feel they work well as a team and maintain high standards of patient care. These nurses have fewer colleagues to call upon and immediate specialist consultations are delayed. The skill mix between junior and senior staff also tends to be uneven despite the patient acuity being the same as it is on day shifts and there is a lack of professional development and access to counselling after hours.

Conclusion

While very little empirical knowledge is available on the embodied ways of being, thinking and acting that are at the heart of many nursing rituals and private discussions – overshadowed as they are by the more objective, credible and dominant discourses of logical-rationalism and evidence-based practice – exploring these experiences may be an important way to illuminate the intricate practices of nursing and how this impacts on job satisfaction, evaluations of self-worth and, ultimately, nursing identity. Today, there is an increasing acknowledgement in nursing of the value of the unique and subjective. As health care is currently constituted, science has precedence over religion and spirituality in the clinical world. In the contemporary academy and research field, science is also judged to be more useful to practice than the arts and storytelling. But stories, intuitions, rituals and beliefs in ephemeral aspects about the world – such as soul and spirit – offer a powerful sense of meaning in peoples' lives, and if nursing is about the support of hope and optimism as adjuncts to wellbeing (Rook and Coombs, 2016), then spirituality and the preservation of the sacred are vital to nursing's practice and identity. As Yashinsky (2006) maintains, ghost stories serve an important function in health care – they offer a way to acknowledge spirituality and mystery in the clinical world. Thus, when nurses journey into the unknown and the uncanny with their night shift rituals of shared ghost storytelling, they may be expressing anxieties about power and responsibility, and these stories and their telling may also be manifestations of protest against the marginalisation of spirituality and unique patient experiences in health care. In essence, this storytelling preserves the intuition that is so important in nursing, and provides a way for a long-silenced part of health care to be articulated and heard.

References

Agrillo C (2011) Near-death experience: Out-of-body and out-of-brain? *Review of General Psychology* 15(1): 1–10.

Balaguero J (dir) (2005) *Fragile*. Film. Spain: Castelao Productions.

Barr W (2000) Lunacy revisited: The influence of the moon on mental health and quality of life *Journal of Psychosocial Nursing and Mental Health Service* 38: 28–35.

Bayley S (2015) *If Asylum Walls Could Speak: A Memoir of 50 Years of Mental Health Nursing at Glenside*. Bloomington: Xlibris.

Beck C (2011) Secondary traumatic stress in nurses: A systematic review *Archives Of Psychiatric Nursing* 25(1): 1–10.

Beebe D, Chang J, Kress K and Mattfeldt-Beman M (2017) Diet quality and sleep quality among day and night shift nurses *Journal of Nursing Management* 25(7): 549–557.

Benner P, Tanner C and Chesla C (2009) *Expertise in Nursing Practice: Caring, Clinical Judgment, and Ethics*. 2nd ed. New York: Springer.

Bennett A and Royle N (2016) *An Introduction to Literature, Criticism and Theory*. London: Routledge.

Betters R (2014) *Nursing's Spookiest Ghost Stories: Haunted Hospitals, Possessed Patients, and Other Tales of Ghostly Health Care Happenings*. Amazon Kindle.

Bern-Klug M (2011) Rituals in nursing homes *Generations: Journal of the American Society on Aging* 35(3): 57–63.

Betty L (2006) Are they hallucinations or are they real? The spirituality of deathbed and near-death visions *Omega* 53: 37–49.

Books C, Coody L, Kauffman R and Abraham S (2017) Night shift work and its health effects on nurses *The Health Care Manager* 36(4): 347–353.

Bosanquet A (2001) Are more babies born in the full moon? The lunar cycle and the onset of labour *MIDIRS Midwifery Digest* 11(1): 61–64.

Bowen M (2018) Family reaction to death. In Titelman P and Reed S K eds *Death and Chronic Illness in the Family*. Abingdon: Routledge, 33–50.

Braun M, Gordon D and Uziely B (2010) Associations between oncology nurses' attitudes toward death and caring for dying patients *Oncology Nursing Forum* 37(1): E43–49.

Brayne S, Lovelace H and Fenwick P (2008) End-of-life experiences and the dying process in a Gloucestershire nursing home as reported by nurses and care assistants *American Journal of Hospice and Palliative Medicine* 25(3): 195–206.

Briggs J (2012) The ghost story. In Punter D (ed) *A New Companion to the Gothic*. London: Wiley, 176–185.

Brixius L, Dunsky E and Wallem L (creators) (2009–2015) *Nurse Jackie*. Television series. Hollywood: Showtime.

Brown R and Brooks I (2002) Emotion at work: Identifying the emotional climate of night nursing *Journal of Management in Medicine* 16(5): 327–344.

Carter M (2009) Trust, power, and vulnerability: A discourse on helping in nursing *Nursing Clinics* 44(4): 393–405.

Cho E, Lee N, Kim E, Kim S, Lee K, Park K and Sung Y (2016) Nurse staffing level and overtime associated with patient safety, quality of care, and care left undone in hospitals: A cross-sectional study. *International Journal of Nursing Studies* 60: 263–271.

Cleary M, Dean S, Sayers J and Jackson D (2018) Nursing and stereotypes *Issues in Mental Health Nursing* 39(2): 192–194.

Cowling III W, Smith M and Watson J (2008) The power of wholeness, consciousness, and caring a dialogue on nursing science, art, and healing *Advances in Nursing Science* 31(1): E41–51.

Dawson A, Stasa H, Roche M, Homer C and Duffield C (2014) Nursing churn and turnover in Australian hospitals: Nurses' perceptions and suggestions for supportive strategies *BMC Nursing* 13(1): 1–10.

Donahue P (2011) *Nursing, The Finest Art: An Illustrated History*. New York: Mosby.

Fenwick P and Brayne S (2011) End-of-life experiences: Reaching out for compassion, communication, and connection-meaning of deathbed visions and coincidences *American Journal of Hospice and Palliative Medicine* 28(1): 7–15.

Foster R and Roenneberg T (2008) Human responses to the geophysical daily, annual and lunar cycles *Current Biology* 18(17): R784–794.

Freud S (1957) Repression. In Freud S (ed) *The Standard Edition of the Complete Psychological Works of Sigmund Freud, Volume XIV (1914–1916): On the History of the Psycho-Analytic Movement, Papers on Metapsychology and Other Works*. London: Hogarth Press, 141–158. Originally published 1915.

Garcez A (2013) *Ghost Stories of the Medical Profession*. New Mexico: Red Rabbit Press.

Gough A (2011) Modern-day ghostbusters suiting up with array of paranormal-sniffing gadgetry. *The Sunday Mail* (Qld) 7 August. Available at: www.couriermail.com.au/news/modern-day-ghostbusters-suiting-up-with-array-of-paranormal-sniffing-gadgetry/news-story/6cbed6ce342fd0c0f15a39a056af1700.

Gouthro T (2009) Recognizing and addressing the stigma associated with mental health nursing: A critical perspective *Issues in Mental Health Nursing* 30(11): 669–676.

Grice-Swenson D (2015) *The Culture of Night Nursing*. Garden City: Adelphi University.

Grundmann C (1990) Proclaiming the gospel by healing the sick?: Historical and theological annotations on medical mission *International Bulletin of Mission Research* 14(3): 120–126.

History B (2010) Haunted places and ghost stories of Brisbane Qld. *Brisbane History*. Available at: www.brisbanehistory.com/ghosts_of_brisbane.html.

Horner A and Zlosnik S (2016) No country for old women: gender, age and the Gothic. In Horner A and Zlosnik S (eds). *Women and the Gothic: An Edinburgh Companion*. Edinburgh: Edinburgh University Press, 184.

Hughes S (2015) Out with vampires, in with haunted houses: The ghost story is back. *The Guardian*. Available at: www.theguardian.com/books/2015/oct/24/out-with-vampires-in-with-haunted-houses-ghost-stories-are-back.

Jones A and Kelly D (2014) Deafening silence? Time to reconsider whether organisations are silent or deaf when things go wrong *BMJ Quality and Safety* 23(9): 709–713.

Kristeva J (1982) *The Powers of Horror: An Essay on Abjection*. Trans. Leon Roudiez. New York: Columbia University Press.

Ladd C, Grimley K, Hickman C and Touhy T (2013) Teaching end-of-life nursing using simulation *Journal of Hospice and Palliative Nursing* 15(1): 41–51.

Laredo J (2018) 'Horror occupied her mind': Misinformation, Misperception, and the Trauma of Gothic Heroines *Aeternum* 5(2): 68–79.

Lin P, Chen C, Pan S, Chen Y, Pan C, Hung H and Wu M (2015) The association between rotating shift work and increased occupational stress in nurses *Journal of Occupational Health* 57(4): 307–315.

Litvak A (dir) (1948) *The Snake Pit*. Film. Hollywood: 20th Century Fox.

Lorenza G, Claudia C, Patrizia M and Valerio D (2017) Caring for dying patient and their families *Journal of Palliative Care* 32(3–4): 127–133.

Margot J (2015) No evidence of purported lunar effect on hospital admission rates or birth rates *Nursing Research* 64(3): 168–175.

Marks I (1969) *Fears and Phobias*. New York: Academic Press.

McAllister M (2017) "Fragile": An examination of the nurse as gothic trope and its significance in today's turbulent world of health care *Aeternum: The Journal of Contemporary Gothic Studies* 4(1): 59–72.

McAllister M and Brien D L (2019) Creatures of the night: Investigating nursing ghost stories. *Aeternum: The Journal of Contemporary Gothic Studies* 6(1). Available at: www.aeternumjournal.com/issues.

Nelson S (2007) Embodied Knowing?: The Constitution of Expertise as Moral Practice in Nursing. *Texto & Contexto-Enfermagem* 16 (1): 136–141.

Owens M and McGowan I W (2006) Madness and the moon: the lunar cycle and psychopathology. *German Journal of Psychiatry* 9(1): 123–127.

Papantoniou K, Devore E, Massa J, Strohmaier S, Vetter C, Yang L, Shi Y, Giovannucci E, Speizer F and Schernhammer E (2018) Rotating night shift work and colorectal cancer risk in the nurses' health studies *International Journal of Cancer* 143(11): 2709–2717.

Piatti-Farnell L (2017) Gothic reflections: Mirrors, mysticism, and cultural hauntings in contemporary horror film *Australasian Journal of Popular Culture* 6(2): 179–194.

Piatti-Farnell L (2018) Cyber-hauntings: The online ghost story and its cultural narratives. In Brewster S and Thurston L eds *The Routledge Handbook to the Ghost Story*. London: Routledge, 397–406.

Piatti-Farnell and Brien D L eds. (2015) *New Directions in 21st-century Gothic: The Gothic Compass*. London: Routledge.

Redding E (2016) 49 Real nurses share the terrifying hospital ghost stories that scared them to death. *Thought Catalog*. Available at: https://thoughtcatalog.com/eric-redding/2016/02/49-real-nurses-tell-the-terrifying-hospital-ghost-stories-that-scared-them-to-death.

Reimer-Kirkham S, Sharma S, Pesut B, Sawatzky R, Meyerhoff H and Cochrane M (2012) Sacred spaces in public places: Religious and spiritual plurality in health care *Nursing Inquiry* 19(3): 202–212.

Rook H and Coombs M (2016) Giving voice to optimism and hope for the future of nursing *Collegian* 23(4): 397–398.

Royle N (2003) *The Uncanny*. Manchester and New York: Manchester University Press.

Sandelowski M (1994) We are the stories we tell: Narrative knowing in nursing practice *Journal of Holistic Nursing* 12(1): 23–33.

Silveira M, Camponogara S and Beck C (2016) Scientific production about night shift work in nursing: A review of literature *Revista De Pesquisa: Cuidado É Fundamental Online* 8(1): 3679–3690.

Smith K (2018) 8 Ghost Stories as Shared by Nurses. Blog. Accessed February 23, 2019. https://nurseslabs.com/8-ghost-stories-shared-nurses.

Snelson A (2004) Under the Brighton full moon *Mental Health Practice* 8(4): 30–34.

Spooner C (2006) *Contemporary Gothic*. London: Reaktion Books.

Steffck (2016) What's your best nursing ghost story? *All Nurses* 1 November. Available at: http://allnurses.com/general-nursing-discussion/whats-your-best-108202.html.

Stillwell B (2004) *Danvers State: Memoirs of a Nurse in the Asylum*. Bloomington: AuthorHouse.

Tahghighi M, Rees C, Brown J, Breen L and Hegney D (2017) What is the impact of shift work on the psychological functioning and resilience of nurses?: An integrative review *Journal of Advanced Nursing* 73(9): 2065–2083.

Watson C (2019) *The Language of Kindness: A Nurse's Story*. London: Chatto and Windus.

Wiese M, Stancliffe R, Read S, Jeltes G and Clayton J (2015) Learning about dying, death, and end-of-life planning: Current issues informing future actions *Journal of Intellectual and Developmental Disability* 40(2): 230–235.

Woolf V (1966) The supernatural in fiction. *Times Literary Supplement*. 31 January 1918. In Woolf L ed *Collected Essays by Virginia Woolf, Vol.1*. London: Hogarth Press, 293–296.

Wright D and Brajtman S (2011) Relational and embodied knowing: Nursing ethics within the interprofessional team *Nursing Ethics* 18(1): 20–30.

Yashinsky D (2006) *Suddenly They Heard Footsteps: Storytelling for the Twenty-first Century*. Jackson: University Press of Mississippi.

Zizek S (2009) *First as Tragedy, Then as Farce*. London: Verso.

6 Mighty, mean, monstrous nurses

Introduction

Popular culture is replete with representations of nurses who are intimidating, manipulative and wily, and even those who are dangerously unhinged. Such transgressive depictions are a significant subversion of the cultural stereotype of the nurse as caring, demure and good. As previously discussed, the good nurse trope – the assumption that all nurses are demure and inherently driven to altruistically care – is an essentialised and simplistic image (Gordon and Nelson, 2006), but is so widely accepted that its transgression makes for powerful storytelling. The nurse character in such transgressive narratives may be a "battleaxe"; capable and knowledgeable but imaged as dominant and domineering. Or, a nurse character may be monstrously cruel, insane or the epitome of evil. This chapter focuses on nurse characters where their flaws are extreme and located in the realm of the grotesque. These are the fictional nurses made memorable due to the way they cunningly use their knowledge and power to effect nefarious outcomes. These are nurses who are mean and monstrous. Considering the representations of "bad" nurses in this way – not all of whom are women – is instructive as it reveals a series of paradoxes associated with nursing's image and identity.

When such nurse characters are female, they epitomise Creed's conceptualisation of the monstrous-feminine (1993) – women who are feared not only because of their power and expert knowledge, but also due to their female gender. Creed argues that, within Western societies, a strong patriarchal ideology still prevails, and this involves a deep-seated fear of women's strength and power. As a result, men and male-dominated societies or cultures need to reclaim dominance by representing strong female characters as monsters who effectively castrate the male characters. This does not mean there are not malevolent male nurses in popular culture but, in terms of monstrous nurses in popular culture, the female variety does predominate both in terms of numbers of representations and how iconic they have become in public imagination.

Such an analysis is relevant to nursing in Western societies, as it became a predominantly female occupation in the nineteenth century. This was partly as a result of the efforts of various European Protestant organisations, such as the Kaiserswerth Deaconess Institute in Germany that established centres of care for thousands of vulnerable people, including children and the elderly and poor. Along with these benevolent services, the Institute established a School of Nursing for Protestant deaconesses, its most famous graduate being Florence Nightingale (Houweling, 2004). Since then, the struggles and achievements of the nursing profession have closely paralleled those of women. The ways nurses and nursing have been represented in popular culture and the mass media have similarly changed over this time, reflecting these struggles and achievements, as well as the various reactions these changes in women's status have engendered. The chapter, therefore, considers the social forces that constrain, influence and inspire nursing's identity, using ideas drawn from feminism, including psychoanalytic feminism.

Effects of the feminist movement

In the early 1980s, the US television series *Nurse* (1981–1982) was popular across many countries. The series followed a telemovie of the same title (1980), both of which were adapted from the bestselling biographical book also titled *Nurse* (Anderson, 1979). This volume was based on a series of interviews with a nurse in Philadelphia, and written, its author Peggy Anderson stated, to reveal the realities of nursing, which she characterised as "grueling, conflicted, undervalued and immensely gratifying" (qtd. in Roberts, 2016; online). Scriptwriter Sue Grafton, later and best known for her much-loved "alphabet series" of crime novels featuring private eye Kinsey Millhone (published 1982–2017), first wrote the telemovie and then the series, which both focused on an attractive, mature woman, Mary Benjamin. This lead was played by Michael Learned, who was well-known for having then most recently played the mother, Olivia Walton, in popular television series *The Waltons* (Hamner, 1972–1979). In *Nurse*, Benjamin returns to work as a supervising nurse in a city hospital after her husband dies, each episode following the dual plotlines of her life as a single woman and being a team leader working with challenging patient and staff issues in a busy New York hospital. This is foreshadowed in the opening sequence of the telemovie, which begins with the Benjamin family at leisure. While the father and son play tennis, wife and mother Mary wins at cards. When her husband collapses, Mary is shown as, at first, personally devastated, and then – within a moment – professionally competently in charge of the situation, performing chest compressions on her husband's prone figure and directing the mouth-to-mouth resuscitation. Once she returns to the work that she had given up some twenty years before when she married, Mary must deal with both the challenges of the demanding medical cases in her charge and the sexism of the doctors with whom she works. Meeting these trials, Mary is shown to effectively harness the forms of nursing knowledge explored in the previous chapter. She is both technically effective and compassionate and intuitive in her role. In terms of portraying high levels of nursing responsibility and competence and showing how the work of the nurse was essential, and complementary, to that of the doctors, all three elaborations of the *Nurse* story – book, telemovie and series – offer a progressive view of nursing.

The series, however, also reveals the paradoxes of feminism's (and women's) achievements at this time. On the one hand, women could enjoy intellectually challenging and rewarding careers, yet they continued to battle sexism and paternalism both at work and in the personal sphere. While this situation has developed since the 1980s, chauvinistic attitudes and gender discrimination have continued in health care, as in society more generally and, for the predominantly female profession of nursing, this can mean seeing advancement as taking two steps forward and one step back (Burke, 2005). For nurses (as, again, for women), emancipation and actualisation has progressed, but is still incomplete.

Mighty "battleaxe" nurses

Perhaps the most recognisable example of the "mean nurse" stereotype in popular culture can be described as the "battleaxe" – a nurse-leader who is unattractive, unempathic and impatient. Perhaps stemming from a fear of women in leadership positions (Gutek, 1985; Oakley, 2000), "she" (for, despite a very small number of exceptions such as Matron Hilary Loftus in *Getting On*, as discussed in Chapter 1, this nurse is almost exclusively female) sets high, and sometimes unachievable, standards. Her powerful presence and deep knowledge base earn her (often begrudging) respect, but also leads to her being feared by both those who work with her and her patients. These nursing characters are compelling and make for gripping and popular stories. A list of just some of the films and television series in which the battleaxe nurse appears reveals how repeatedly the stereotype has been utilised, as well as the wide range of genres of stories in which it appears: *Shock* (Werker, 1946), *The Snake Pit* (Litvak, 1948), *The Young Doctors* (Watson, 1973–1983), *One Flew Over the Cuckoo's Nest* (Forman, 1975), *High Anxiety* (Brooks, 1977), *Misery* (Reiner, 1990), *Fragile* (Balaguero, 2005), *Psychoville* (Lipsey, 2009-2011), *Shutter Island* (Scorsese, 2010), *The Ward* (Carpenter, 2010) and *Crimson Field* (Clark, Evans and O'Sullivan, 2014). An actual battle axe is a deadly weapon designed to be used in medieval warfare (Nicholson, 2004). Unlike the axe used for wood-cutting, the battle axe was carved from iron or steel and designed to sever limbs with one stroke and vanquish opponents. When transferred to refer to forceful women, and then to forceful (usually female) nurses, the term is consistently used pejoratively.

In *Carry on Nurse* (Thomas, 1959), women are in charge, and the male patients are potentially at their mercy. In 1959, this was generally understood as a situation rich in comedic potential due to its subversion of the reality of life at this time. This also serves as a backdrop for sexist jokes and general mayhem. In this topsy-turvy version of the world of a hospital, a glimpse of a nurse's shapely seamed stockinged legs leads to drooling and nudging amongst the male patients. Sometimes, such subversion includes men donning the nursing uniform, as occurs, for example, in *Carry On Doctor* (Thomas, 1967). But the matron in charge, who is buxom and formidable, evokes a much different reaction. Patients whisper to each other in her presence and are shown to be tremblingly afraid. In one scene, in the middle of her round, she is confronted by a disgruntled patient, Mr. Reckitt. He sees no reason for her strict rule about patients not remaining in their beds unless they are sick and decides to challenge her. Mockingly, he asks her, "So it's not a *medical* rule?" The matron, appalled at his challenge, replies that she does not see what that has to do with it, implying that it is *her* rule. Mr Reckitt answers in a patronising tone:

> I'll explain, Matron. If a doctor asks me to hang by one arm from the ceiling wearing an aqualung … I'll do it! He aims to cure me. Your rule has nothing to do with my cure, therefore it has no meaning.

When the shocked Matron tries to protest, Reckitt dismisses her, saying he wants to rest. The matron is struck dumb and, still appalled, stamps off, leading to fearfully exchanged glances amongst the nurses. They know that repercussions for them will ensue because her will has been thwarted. In this scene, the matron is the binary opposite – in appearance, demeanour and appeal – of the young and slender clinical nurses on the ward, and this is played on for comic effect throughout the film. In the normal scheme of things, nurses represent trustworthiness, safety and stability; but when the world is not functioning correctly, these expectations are dashed and comedy (or drama) results.

The battleaxe matron's subversion of the good nurse stereotype, plus the tension generated between women (nurses and matron), as featured in this film are well-used narrative devices in hospital comedies and dramas. As a counterpoint to the demure nurse stereotype, the battleaxe matron represents everything that the "ministering angel" is not. Stern, decisive, independent, unempathic and, often, overweight and asexual, the battleaxe matron is mocked and derided and, in this way, the image of the good nurse – she who is docile, gentle, servile and pretty – is reinforced as the ideal for the public (who are also patients and their carers) as well as nurses themselves. In these narratives, the matron – as a leader and manager – has greater knowledge and influence, and can control events more, than nurses, but she is also feared and is avoided where possible. While a matron's competence is usually not questioned, their lacking personal attributes and strident communication style are harshly emphasised, such that they are personally and professionally derided and their achievements rendered invisible.

Monstrous nurses

The "mean" or "battleaxe nurse" can also become monstrous. A vivid example of this is Nurse Noakes in David Mitchell's novel, *Cloud Atlas* (2004). Nurse Noakes is the authoritarian and vicious head nurse of a nursing home that the novel's protagonist, Timothy Cavendish, thinks is a hotel. Soon realising that he has been imprisoned, for there are locked doors and no windows, Cavendish tries to escape. Nurse Noakes takes sadistic pleasure in caning him for his attempt, her cruelty subsequently inducing a stroke which renders him more docile. Cavendish eventually does escape, and the police are notified with the implication that Noakes will be arrested. The plotline follows the battleaxe nurse trope, with domineering behaviour triggering conflict, which leads to retaliation until order can be restored. In this way, the nurses in such narratives are also portrayed as reproducing and reinforcing – with damaging effect – the dominant masculinised hegemony. Paradoxically, this dynamic reinforces nursing's disempowerment and marginalisation. To be liked, nurses need to be pretty and docile. To be influential, they need to deny their full personhood and embody a parodical version of a powerful and sexless woman. Underscoring this point, Noakes was played in the film version of *Cloud Atlas* (2012) by a man; a towering and ghastly Hugo Weaving who, wearing a "fat suit", blonde wig, lurid makeup and loose white uniform with beige cardigan, says he played her like an "S&M version of Nurse Ratched ... like a monster" (Hochberg, 2012). This works well in the film as the mean and monstrous nurse exists in potent contrast to the good nurse.

Misery, written by Stephen King (1987), and brought to film by Rob Reiner (1990), is a psychological thriller that draws upon the quintessential dramatic trope of the "bad nurse" – a narrative trope that stands in stark contrast with the more prevailing stereotype that all nurses are good. In the film, in the midst of a snowstorm, Nurse Annie Wilkes single-handedly extracts the badly injured novelist, Paul Sheldon, from his crashed car and resuscitates him using cardiac compressions and mouth-to mouth oxygenation. She then carries him to the remote, isolated farmhouse where she lives alone. Wilkes resets Sheldon's fractured limbs, and stabilises him using intravenous fluids, pain relief and careful positioning. Throughout his long recovery, Sheldon is grateful for her attention. When, however, Wilkes insists that Sheldon resumes his writing, the mutuality and comfort in the relationship takes a sickening turn as she transforms from passive reader to "merciless editor" (p. 98) and, slowly but relentlessly, is revealed as more and more unhinged. Her attention becomes more and more obsessive and her nursing becomes callous and dysfunctional.

Wilkes is, thus, a paradox in terms of the commonly held expectations of the selfless nurse (Morgan, 2014), as she transforms from angel to demon when her own desires are unrequited. In *Misery,* the power of the "bad nurse" image can be understood as succeeding, at least in part, because of how vividly viewers expect a nurse to be a figure of angelic, motherly care. Nurse Wilkes, instead, epitomises the notion of Creed's monstrous feminine (1993). Her expert knowledge gives her complete power over the patient and, because she is a woman (and obsessive, irrational and hysterical), this knowledge – which first saved the patient's life – becomes dangerous and destructive. This is in line with Dawson's (1968) classic discussion of paradox

in the Gothic novel, which describes how Gothic texts often emphasise irreconcilable dichotomies and contradictions. Wilkes is, for instance, so skilled
in setting Sheldon's complex fractures that a surgeon is not needed, yet she
has previously been on trial for patient negligence. Instead of being reliable,
calm and selflessly able to deliver Sheldon the care he needs – as in the
stereotypical image of the perfect nurse (Davis, 1992) – she is erratic, selfish
and driven by her own desires. Thus, while caring for Sheldon, she terrifies
him into doing her will.

Wilkes' female gender potentiates her monstrosity. To indicate the extremity of her depravity, readers/viewers learn that she is a serial killer of mater-
nity ward babies, and it is suggested that her motivation for this horrendous
crime may be to exact revenge against the world for her own childlessness.
In another example of her lack of traditional feminine qualities, Wilkes
threatens Sheldon's masculinity, both explicitly in terms of her threat to castrate him, and implicitly in her control of him. As Wilkes loses both her feminine decorum and her grip on reality, Sheldon, recovering his sense of
masculinity, stops thinking as a passive patient and begins to plot his escape.
As Sheldon's health improves, Wilkes' malevolence grows, and the story
reaches its climax when Wilkes discovers his plan. In a horrific parody of
nursing communication, she matter-of-factly explains that he is about to be
"hobbled" – an abhorrent operation once performed to keep slaves from
escaping but still able to work (Richardson and Locks, 2014). In the ultimate
perversion of nursing professionalism, as Sheldon begins to scream, she tells
him she loves him, and he finally understands that to survive her insane min-
istrations, he must adopt her murderous techniques. A vital dynamic between
these two characters, and one that heightens the horror of the narrative of
both novel and film is, thus, the patient-nurse relationship between the
story's two principal characters, and how the nurse's care, once it changes
into a perverted form of obsessive love, becomes twisted into aberrant and
damaging torture.

In Wilkes' extreme transgression of what is expected of a nurse, the reader/
viewer of *Misery* feels a measure of the fear, and even horror and terror, that
many real-life patients have reported they have felt at the hands of neglectful and
unkind nurses. Jeffs (2009), for instance, has described the impression of being
controlled and patronised by nursing staff. Other researchers have reported
patients being humiliated and shamed (Karlsson and Forsberg, 2008), and even
violated, terrified and victimised by nurses (Skyman, Sjöström, and Hellström,
2010). Thus, this horror story hyperbolises what is often lying dormant in
patients' minds about what might happen if they encounter an incompetent or
unethical nurse. A major contributor to the global nursing shortage is lack of
professional fulfillment. Numerous authors have argued the need for better
career structures and nurse patient ratios and additional professional support to
offset these concerns (Aiken et al., 2008; McHugh et al., 2011), but less widely
known is the influence that patient dissatisfaction with care has on a nurse's work
self-efficacy. Eriksson and Svedlund (2007) argue that patient satisfaction surveys

communicate very little and more research needs to be undertaken to understand sources of patient dissatisfaction, such as how they come to feel ignored, belittled and excluded. The figure of the monstrous nurse in popular culture is, therefore, of considerable significance as this reveals potent anxieties that often go unnoticed and unexplored in the healthcare context.

Mean and monstrous nurses

Combining ideas of the mean battleaxe and the monstrous nurse is Nurse Ratched, also known as Big Nurse, from *One Flew Over the Cuckoo's Nest* (Kesey, 1962). Nurse Ratched is such a terrifying nurse that she has reached iconic status in popular culture due to both this novel and the film made from it (Forman, 1975). This is partly because she defies simple categorisation. At first glance, and in popular imagination, Nurse Ratched is the epitome of the monstrous nurse – powerful, grim and pitted against her patients. Additionally, unlike Annie Wilkes, Nurse Ratched's actions are veiled and ambiguous, which makes her even more frightening as a character. Ratched is subtly physically attractive and, outwardly, she appears self-contained, and maternal in a protective, calming way; that is, not the typical battleaxe, although she is controlling and feared. An early description from the narrator of the novel (Chief Bromden) suggests that her outward composure and appearance may not correspond with her internal motivations, suggesting an enigmatic complexity:

> She stops and nods at some of the patients come to stand around and stare out of eyes all red and puffy with sleep. She nods one to each. Precise, automatic gesture. Her face is smooth, calculated, and precision-made, like an expensive baby doll, skin like flesh colored enamel, blend of white and cream and baby-blue eyes, small nose, pink little nostrils – everything working together except the color on her lips and fingernails, and the size of her bosom.
>
> (p. 11)

This description indicates that Nurse Ratched's gender is part of the reason why the narrator dislikes her. Other descriptions make her appear cold and emotionless in the face of the distress of patients who, with serious mental illnesses, are incarcerated in a restrictive, soulless environment. She sets the schedule for these patients, probes and challenges their psyches, and approves or disapproves their requests. This can be seen in her carefully modulated controlling response to McMurphy's request that she unlock the day room so that the patients can play cards:

> She smiles and closes her eyes again and shakes her head gently. "Of course, you may take the suggestion up with the rest of the staff at some time, but I'm afraid everyone's feelings will correspond with mine: we do not have adequate

coverage for two day rooms. There isn't enough personnel. And I wish you wouldn't lean against the glass there, please; your hands are oily and staining the window. That means extra work for some of the other men."

He jerks his hand away, and I see he starts to say something and then stops, realizing she didn't leave him anything else to say, unless he wants to start cussing at her. His face and neck are red. He draws a long breath and concentrates on his will power, the way she did this morning, and tells her that he is very sorry to have bothered her, and goes back to the card table.

(p. 87)

Chief Bromden's narration also derides her efficiency and the knowledge she has of all the patients. In this, there is the suggestion that Nurse Ratched, not the forensic mental patients in the institution, is the "Other" in this story, and that this otherness causes profound problems. This is also displayed in her self-containment in the face of chaos, and how she has access to knowledge to which that few others in the setting are privy. The subtle, and quite terrifying, ferocity that she can display also distinguishes her from other battleaxe matrons represented in novels, films and on television, and contributes to making *One Flew Over the Cuckoo's Nest* the memorable classic it has become.

Nurse Ratched's character is also, in part, compelling simply because she defies so many of the taken-for-granted assumptions about nurses. While female, she is not a sex-symbol because she is neither demure nor available. Rather than being caring and empathic, she appears impassive and cold. She is not the nurturing, helpful surrogate mother that the patients (and readers/viewers) expect her to be. Indeed, within this story, it is the male patients who rescue, nurture, inspire and empower each other. McMurphy, for example, himself an incarcerated and damaged man, motivates several of the anxious, ambivalent and powerless patients to take action and, in the process, some control of the situation. This is what Hunter (1988) describes as the "translocated ideal", the psychodynamic process in which an unachieved Oedipal desire is repressed and the ideal mother is transferred and located onto others. Instead of idealising the matron, the men loathe and blame her, while revering McMurphy, the male anti-hero. Munoz (2013) sees this narrative operating as a kind of wish-fulfillment – satisfying an urge that readers/viewers have to answer back to a world that has become strictly authoritarian as well as anti-feminist.

Others note the complexity in her portrayal as a mental health nurse. For Darbyshire (1995), Ratched is a nurse who is under a great deal of pressure, having to care for a large number of forensic mental patients as well as to manage incompetent and malicious staff. The austere system in which she works limits the resources available to the staff, compelling the nurses (led by Ratched) to set strict rules to ensure that every patient is bathed, receives their medications and is at least safe in the frightening space in which they find themselves. Incursions and inhumane actions do occur, but it is mainly Ratched who takes the blame, even though other staff and patients create trouble. For example, the orderlies, are described as brutes.

Most days I'm the first one to see the Admission [McMurphy] watch him creep in the door and slide along the wall and stand scared till the black boys come sign for him and take him into the shower room, where they strip him and leave him shivering with the door open while they all three run grinning up and down the halls looking for the Vaseline. "We need that Vaseline," they'll tell the Big Nurse, "for the thermometer." She looks from one to the other: "I'm sure you do," and hands them a jar that holds at least a gallon, "but mind you boys don't group up in there." Then I see two, maybe all three of them in there, in that shower room with the Admission, running that thermometer around in the grease till it's coated the size of your finger, crooning, "Tha's right, mothah, that's right," and then shut the door and turn all the showers up to where you can't hear anything but the vicious hiss of water on the green tile. I'm out there most days, and I see it like that.

(p. 15)

Kalisch and Kalisch (1987) suggest that, at the superficial level, Ratched is the perfect nurse. She is attractive, calm, commands her team confidently, and ensures the ward runs in an orderly manner. She also shows a high level of commitment since she has dedicated her life to the job and to the male patients. Importantly, Nurse Ratched does show sympathy at times, for example when Billy Bobbit is distressed, she provides comfort. The story continues, however, to criticise the measures she uses, describing how, "She continued to glare at us as she spoke. It was strange to hear that voice, soft and soothing and warm as a pillow, coming out of a face hard as porcelain" (p. 248). Perhaps this is why Munoz (2013) believes Ratched to be offering insincere care and that this idea of insincerity gets to the heart of her malevolence. Munoz writes that a part of her "magnetic presence" is due to "her existence in the world as a person wiling to display a coldly insincere concern that, nevertheless, gets eaten up by the neediest as genuine care" (p. 670).

The novel culminates in an attack on Nurse Ratched that ultimately takes away her power – she is sexually assaulted and humiliated and, as a result, her chimera of self-control is exposed.

Screaming when he grabbed for her and ripped her uniform all the way down the front, screaming again when the two nippled circles started from her chest and swelled out and out, bigger than anybody had ever even imagined, warm and pink in the light – only at last, after the officials realized that the three black boys weren't going to do anything but stand and watch and they would have to beat him off without their help, doctors and supervisors and nurses prying those heavy red fingers out of the white flesh of her throat as if they were her neck bones.

(p. 250)

In this way, Ratched is utterly degraded, her professional and personal persona and identity shattered. Kesey's story positions her as the head nurse and representative of a harsh, unwielding institution but, as she does to McMurphy, she also represents women's oppression of men (Darbyshire, 1995), symbolic of the disastrous consequences that occur when men lose their masculinity (Muñoz, 2013). So not only is this nurse-in-charge dangerous because of her legitimate power, she is dangerous because her sexual potency threatens all the surrounding men. This threat illustrates the concept of the backlash against feminism, as elucidated by Faludi (2009). The feminist backlash is important to consider in this context because it explains the historic, and ongoing, struggle for women – and for nursing as a predominantly female profession (Sullivan, 2002) – against institutionalised and culturally embedded sexism.

The barriers for nursing's advancement are political and cultural. Gender inequality locks nursing into a lower status. MacWilliams et al. (2013) argues that nursing remains predominantly a profession for women. Men are still not actively encouraged to enter nursing, and in some countries are actively discouraged, even though equality benefits individuals as well as society (MacWilliams, Schmidt and Bleich, 2013). Nurses, many of whom are (like Nurse Jackie) the primary caregivers in their family, often endure a "double day" of work – in their hospital role, and then at home with childcare, cooking, cleaning, shopping and other domestic responsibilities. No other profession requires so little education for so much responsibility (Sullivan, 2002). Although the fight for degree-level education for nursing benefits nurses and patients, there are still many in society (Templeton, 2004) who think that nursing was better when students were less bent on what has been called their "quest for professional recognition" (Corbin, 2008, 164). They argue that when nurses become adept at technical and complex procedures their ability (and presumably willingness) to care is lessened.

This is, however, simplistic because, when patients need highly technical and curative care – such as when they are in acute biological crisis – their need for caring is also at its highest (Griffiths, 2008). It is not possible to separate these two needs, and so it remains a legitimate goal for nurses to be capable of exercising both technical and carative supports to patients at the same time. Further, the claim that nurses prefer the technical over the carative aspects of their work could well be a diversionary tactic to avoid acknowledgement that managerialism and economic rationalism prioritises care that can be measured and overlooks care that is more affective, and thus not easily measured. Nurses are not happy with this situation and, indeed, numerous studies have repeatedly identified that nurses do not surrender their caring ideals, but instead feel they are blocked and undermined by policy and that these are the sources for their disillusionment (Johnson, 2018; Maben, Latter and Macleod Clark, 2007; Sharp, McAllister and Broadbent, 2017). Thus, it is not nurses who devalue caring, but society (Maben, 2008). Caring is, in a sense, invisible and is not missed, until it is gone. This axiom is evident and emphasised in *One Flew over the Cuckoo's Nest* and following this line of argument offers another way to read Nurse Ratched. That is, to understand that she does perform callous acts that lead to patient harm, but to also comprehend that she may not be solely responsible for these actions. As Bloom (2000) argues, social service systems and the staff working within them are frequently traumatised by a phenomenon explained as "parallel processes". This occurs in mental health services due to:

> Complex interactions between traumatized clients, stressed staff, pressured organizations, and a social and economic environment that is frequently hostile to the aims of recovery, [with the result that] our systems frequently recapitulate the very experiences that have proven to be so toxic for the people we are supposed to treat.
>
> (p. 13)

All these actions and interactions are evident within the environment portrayed in both the novel, and filmed version of, *One Flew Over the Cuckoo's Nest*. Reading these texts, and the nurses within them through this lens, calls into question where the cause of the dysfunction lies. In such a reading, both the book and the film function as treatises exposing the consequences of totalitarian institutions. As works of art that have stood the test of time, novel and film are also expositions on how psychiatry has long struggled to balance the social demands of confinement with the humanistic aspirations of care (Clarke, 2009).

These narratives affect readers and viewers in another important way – voicing a fear that many people have about going to hospital, and the treatment they will receive there. This issue is even more complex in relation to psychiatric treatment, as there remains a stigma about mental illness. Many people believe the myths that a diagnosis of a mental disorder will be a lifelong sentence, and that such an illness is synonymous with *losing one's mind* (Overton and Medina, 2008). Many believe that people with mental illness are all erratic, impulsive or violent (Feldman and Crandall, 2007). These fears regarding mental illness also extend towards psychiatric health professionals and mental health care facilities, and explains why many people are afraid of, and want to avoid hospitalisation (Schulze, 2007).

Nurses themselves struggle with Ratched's portrayal and notoriety. A number of advocacy groups and researchers (see Stanley, 2008, 2012) have questioned the way nursing is portrayed in the media, and their studies always include mention of Ratched. The American-based media watchdog, *The Truth about Nursing*, voiced opposition to a plan by Netflix to produce a television series that imagines her character's earlier life and, presumably, explains her rise to power and infamy. Titled simply *Ratched*, the series draws on the popularity of the series *American Horror Story*, indicating its approach. Opponents to the project see this development as reigniting and underscoring an anti-nurse stereotype, and warn that it will have dangerous consequences, including dissuading potential new recruits from joining the profession and exacerbating the worldwide shortage of nurses. Yet, the trope of the mean and monstrous nurse that occurs so repeatedly in popular culture, and which Ratched epitomises, is important to consider. On one level, underscoring these nurses' bad behaviours, such narratives project a view about nursing leaders that they cannot (and, therefore, should not) be trusted with power or knowledge. This is a sexist discourse that is rarely deconstructed. Examination of such narratives reveals an unconscious Oedipal complex in play – unable to claim the mother/nurse as lover, the protagonist finds ways to attack and demean her. This is because narratives that feature nurses in positions of power and influence threaten the status quo. In order for the patriarchy to reclaim this lost power, and for the "natural order" to be restored, the nurse must reduced in some way, often to her flawed sexuality, which therefore makes *her* position (as nurses' sexuality is overwhelmingly portrayed as feminine) worthless, waning and trivial. On another level, these narratives can be read metaphorically. When a nurse character is endowed with too much power, control and influence, surpassing what any "normal" individual ought to possess, as well as overriding the systemic safeguards, this can be read as a criticism of the entire health care system. Any systems that allows unchecked omnipotence are likely to become dysfunctional, oppressing the people they are meant to serve, and falling inexorably into entropy.

Real nurses acting badly

There are, of course, cases where real nurses have acted as mean or monstrously as the figures in these fictions. When nurses are found to have transgressed against the standards of professional behaviour, they are rightly subjected to scrutiny and, when warranted, professional and/or legal censure. A potent example of this is American conman and sociopath John Meehan. Losing his license as a nurse anaesthetist after he took a firearm into an operating theatre, Meehan was discovered to have stolen prescription medications from the hospital in which he worked. He was arrested for this drug theft, but fled from custody and, when apprehended, served additional time in prison for resisting arrest and drug possession. He masqueraded as a medical specialist – an anaesthetist – using this respected persona to attract women and fraudulently obtain money from them, including by terrifying acts of abuse and harassment. This callous and disastrous series of events has been characterised as "a reign of terror" (Dibdin, 2019). The story was first disseminated in public in Pullitzer Prize winning journalist Christopher Goffard's investigative true crime podcast series *Dirty John* (2017a) and six associated *LA Times* newspaper stories (Goffard, 2017b, 2017c, 2017d, 2017e, 2017f, 2017g). In a matter of weeks from its release, this podcast series had become wildly popular with millions of downloads in the USA, Australia, Canada and the UK and was later made into an eponymous dramatised television series using actors (Cunningham, 2018) and also a documentary *Dirty John: The Dirty Truth* (Mast, 2019). Unlike the fictitious characters so far examined,

Meehan's motivations may have been even more abhorrent than that of Ratched or Wilkes – for, at least, they appeared to have begun their nursing careers with benevolent intent. Meehan, instead, saw nursing as an opportunity to exploit vulnerable people and to access what he greedily desired – drugs and money. What such real-life monsters and those brought to life on screen share is the common aspect of being terrifying examples of a caring profession corrupted to its core.

Complexities of care

These narratives of real, and fictional, failures of nursing caring in popular culture, are illuminating. This is because there remains a deep-seated ambivalence towards care in society. Caring is complex, and difficult. While lip service is easily paid to the importance of caring, it is not easily talked about in depth or fostered. Yet it is deeply connected to human nature, and, as such – and given the "good nurse" trope – it is easy to make the mistake of thinking that in nursing, care must come naturally. When it does not, or when it is thwarted, rather than assess the conditions surrounding nurses in their working day, nurses themselves are attacked. The "too posh to wash" criticism made familiar in the British press (Chapman, 2013), which censures nurses for not performing what are seen as their core duties, can be read not only as professional criticism, but evidence of a backlash against nursing's educational progress and projection of blame for austere management policies. This is not to suggest that some nurses may well deserve to be confronted and contained. Others, though, may be collateral damage as society refuses to acknowledge its own role in devaluing care.

While nursing as a profession is evolving alongside the scientific, social and technical revolutions that are affecting health care and the health care system, these revolutions have not been entirely positive for nurses and nursing. The medical science revolution has, for instance, been momentous for nursing because it has led to specialties in nursing developing, each with its own discrete sets of knowledge, interventions, educational programmes and career pathways. This process of specialisation has also, however, been blamed for fracturing nursing by exacerbating competition for scarce medical and educational resources (Hutchinson et al., 2006), and promoting a hierarchy of specialisations, with some valorised (such as emergency and paediatric nursing) and others (such as psychiatry and aged care) stigmatised (McCann, Clark and Lu, 2010). Advances in medicine and the advent of specialisations, have also, in part, led to increased levels of education for nurses. Social revolutions, particularly feminism, have assisted in the professionalisation of nursing, elevating the standard of education and training available so that nursing is now on a par with other responsible occupations like teaching and law. Despite improvement in education, wages and conditions, however, nursing continues to be understood by many as a manual, working class career (Carpenter, 2018) and needed structural changes such as revised nurse/patient ratios, permanent employment and adequate recompense for shift work have still not occurred in most parts of the health services (Bogossian, Winters-Chang and Tuckett, 2014). The public have little tolerance for ongoing protests or the possibility of nurses striking en masse and, as a result, improvements in working conditions have been localised and piecemeal (Sasso et al., 2017; Trinkoff et al., 2006).

Conclusion

In popular culture, the development of a transgressive counter-narrative to the "good nurse" has proliferated. In the post-war period, this can be conjectured to be, at least in part, because of the backlash against women's new-found public status and access to power, as well as a reaction to the politics, and achievements, of feminism. Revealing something of patient anxieties, the compelling image of the mean or monstrous nurse – someone who exploits their knowledge and power for malicious, malevolent intent, or has incorrect (and elevated) ideas about what nursing involves – can be analysed for what this imaging reveals about the status of nurses and nursing in society. While many, for instance, read Nurse Ratched as completely cruel, sadistic and unfeeling, she can also, however, be considered as a victim of the system. If read as a cultural symbol for nursing, the figure of Ratched can also reveal some of the hidden paradoxes shaping and constraining how nurses, and nursing, are perceived. Frequently, nurses (both individuals and as a group) are an easy target for attacks against a failing health care system. What is rarely recognised, however, is the extremity of the personal pressures that need to be endured, including the emotions that need to be suppressed, and how compliance with overarching and sometimes dehumanising and unjust policies, in inadequately resourced systems, can be overwhelming. And yet, most nurses continue to tend to the patients and others in their care competently and, often, with care and compassion. Beneath the surface of these actions flow undercurrents of social, class, gender and political divisions that are seldom acknowledged, let alone discussed. Representations in popular culture can not only raise these and other related issues for consideration, but present them in a form in which complex and multiple viewpoints can be discerned and examined.

References

Aiken L, Clarke S, Sloane D, Lake E and Cheney T (2008) Effects of hospital care environment on patient mortality and nurse outcomes *The Journal of Nursing Administration* 38(5): 223–229.

Anderson P (1979) *Nurse: The True Story of Mary Benjamin R.N.* Los Angeles: Berkley.

Balaguero F (dir) (2005) *Fragile*. Film. Barcelona: Filmax.

Bloom S (2000) Creating sanctuary: Healing from systematic abuses of power *Therapeutic Communities: the International Journal for Therapeutic and Supportive Organizations* 21(2): 67–92.

Bogossian F, Winters-Chang P and Tuckett A (2014) "The pure hard slog that nursing is": A qualitative analysis of nursing work *Journal of Nursing Scholarship* 46(5): 377–388.

Brooks M (dir) (1977) *High Anxiety*. Film. Hollywood: Crossbow films.

Burke R (2005) Backlash in the workplace *Women in Management Review* 20(3): 165–176.

Carpenter J (dir) (2010) The Ward. *Film*. London: Filmnation.

Carpenter M (2018) The new managerialism and professionalism in nursing. In, Stacey M, Reid M, Heath C and Dingwall R (eds). *Health and the Division of Labour*. London: Routledge, 165–195.

Chapman J (2013) Nurses told, "you're not too posh to wash a patient": Minister orders student nurses back to basics to improve compassion in NHS. *Daily Mail* 26 March. Available at: www.dailymail.co.uk/news/article–2299085.

Clark R, Evans D and O'Sullivan T (dirs) (2014) *The Crimson Field*. Television series. London: BBC.

Clarke R (2009) The care and confinement of the mentally ill. In Barker P (ed) *Psychiatric and Mental Health Nursing: The Craft of Caring 2nd Ed.* London: Hodder Arnold, 21–29.

Corbin J (2008) Is caring a lost art in nursing? *International Journal of Nursing Studies* 45(2): 163–165.

Creed B (1993) *The Monstrous-Feminine: Film, Feminism, Psychoanalysis*. New York: Routledge.

Cunningham A (creator) (2018) *Dirty John*. Television series. Los Angeles: Bravo.

Darbyshire P (1995) Reclaiming 'Big Nurse': A feminist critique of Ken Kesey's portrayal of Nurse Ratched in *One Flew over the Cuckoo's Nest*. *Nursing Inquiry* 2 (4): 198–202.

Davis C (1992) Nurse as angel of mercy *Literature and Medicine* 11(1): 88–89. https://doi.org/10.1353/lm.2011.0283

Dawson L M (1968) Melmoth the Wanderer: Paradox and the Gothic novel *Studies in English Literature*: 1500–1900, 621–632.

Dibdin E (2019) A complete timeline of the events of "Dirty John": The real-life story is even more shocking than the show. *Harper's Bazaar* 13 January. Available at: www.harpersbazaar.com/culture/film-tv/a25372275/dirty-john-true-story-timeline.

Eriksson U and Svedlund M (2007) Struggling for confirmation: Patients' experiences of dissatisfaction with hospital care *Journal of Clinical Nursing* 16 (3): 438–446.

Faludi S (2009) *Backlash: The Undeclared War Against American Women*. New York: Broadway Books.

Feldman D and Crandall C (2007) Dimensions of mental illness stigma: What about mental illness causes social rejection? *Journal of Social and Clinical Psychology* 26 (2): 137–154.

Forman M dir (1975) *One Flew over the Cuckoo's Nest*. Film Hollywood: Fantasy Films.

Goffard C (2017a) *Dirty John*. Podcast. *Wordery*. Rel. 2–8 October.

Goffard C (2017b) The real thing. *LA Times*, 1 October. Available at: www.latimes.com/projects/la-me-dirty-john.

Goffard C (2017c) Newlyweds. *LA Times*, 2 October. Available at: www.latimes.com/projects/la-me-dirty-john-newlyweds.

Goffard C (2017d) Filthy. *LA Times*, 4 October. Available at: www.latimes.com/projects/la-me-dirty-john-filthy.

Goffard C (2017e) Forgiveness. *LA Times*, 5 October. Available at: www.latimes.com/projects/la-me-dirty-john-forgiveness.

Goffard C (2017f) Escape. *LA Times*, 7 October. Available at: www.latimes.com/projects/la-me-dirty-john-escape.

Goffard C (2017g) Terra. *LA Times*, 8 October. Available at: www.latimes.com/projects/la-me-dirty-john-terra.

Gordon S and Nelson S (2006) Moving beyond the virtue script in nursing: creating a knowledge-based identity for nurses. In Nelson S and Gordon S (eds). *The complexities of care: Nursing reconsidered*. New York: Cornell University Press, 13–29.

Grafton S (creator) (1981–1982) *Nurse*. Television series Hollywood: Viacom.

Griffiths P (2008) The art of losing … ? A response to the question "is caring a lost art?" *International Journal of Nursing Studies* 45(3): 329–332.

Gutek B (1985) *Sex and the Workplace*. San Francisco: Jossey Bass.

Hamner E creator (1972–1979) *The Waltons*. Television series Hollywood: Warner Bros.

Hochberg M (2012) Hugo Weaving on Cloud Atlas, Lana Wachowski, and playing a hefty woman nurse. *Vulture*. Available at: www.vulture.com/2012/09/hugo-weaving-cloud-atlas-interview.html.

Houweling L (2004) Image, function and style: A history of the nursing uniform *American Journal of Nursing* 104(4): 40–48.

Hunter K (1988) Nurses: The satiric image and the translocated ideal. In Jones A (ed) *Images of Nurses: Perspectives from History, Art, and Literature*. Pennsylvania: University of Pennsylvania Press, 113–127.

Hutchinson M, Vickers M, Jackson D and Wilkes L (2006) Workplace bullying in nursing: Towards a more critical organisational perspective *Nursing Inquiry* 13(2): 118–126.

Jeffs S (2009) *Flying with Paper Wings: Reflections on Living with Madness*. Melbourne: Vulgar Press.

Johnson S (2018) "Convince your patients and you will convince society": Career decisions and professional identity among nurses in India. *SAGE Open* 8 March: 1–14.

Kalisch P and Kalisch B (1987) *The Changing Image of the Nurse*. Menlo Park MMenM: Addison-Wesley.

Karlsson V and Forsberg A (2008) Health is yearning: Experiences of being conscious during ventilator treatment in a critical care unit *Intensive and Critical Care Nursing* 24(1): 41–50.

Kesey K (1962) *One Flew Over The Cuckoo's Nest*. London: Pan Books.

King S (1987) *Misery*. London: Hodder & Stoughton.

Lipsey M dir (2009–2011) *Psychoville*. Television series. Mill Hill: BBC.

Litvak A dir (1948) *The Snake Pit*. Film. Hollywood: 20th Century Fox.

Maben J (2008) The art of caring: Invisible and subordinated? A response to Juliet Corbin: "Is caring a lost art in nursing?" *International Journal of Nursing Studies* 45(3): 335–338.

Maben J, Latter S and Macleod Clark J (2007) The challenges of maintaining ideals and standards in professional practice: Evidence from a longitudinal qualitative study *Nursing Inquiry* 14(2): 99–113.

MacWilliams B, Schmidt B and Bleich M (2013) Men in nursing *The American Journal of Nursing* 113(1): 38–44.

Mast S (dir) (2019) *Dirty John: The Dirty Truth*. Television documentary. Los Angeles: Oxygen.

McCann T, Clark E and Lu S (2010) Bachelor of Nursing students' career choices: A three-year longitudinal study *Nurse Education Today* 30(1): 31–36.

McHugh M, Kutney-Lee A, Cimiotti J, Sloane D and Aiken L (2011) Nurses' widespread job dissatisfaction, burnout, and frustration with health benefits signal problems for patient care *Health Affairs* 30(2): 202–210.

Mitchell D (2004) *Cloud Atlas.* London: Random House.

Morgan R (2014) Roy Morgan image of professions survey 2014. Retrieved from www.roymorgan.com, article 5531.

Muñoz M (2013) "A veritable angel of mercy": The problem of Nurse Ratched in Ken Kesey's *One Flew over the Cuckoo's Nest. Southern Review* 49(4): 668–671.

Nicholson H (2004) *Medieval Warfare.* Basingstoke: Palgrave MacMillan.

Oakley J (2000) Gender-based barriers to senior management positions: Understanding the scarcity of female CEOs *Journal of Business Ethics* 27(4): 321–334.

Overton S and Medina S (2008) The stigma of mental illness *Journal of Counseling and Development* 86(2): 143–151.

Reiner R (dir) (1990) *Misery.* Film. Hollywood: Castlerock Entertainment.

Rich D (dir) (1980) *Nurse.* Telemovie. Hollywood: Viacom.

Richardson N and Locks A (2014) *Body Studies: The Basics.* New York: Routledge.

Roberts S (2016) Peggy Anderson, chronicler of the nursing profession, dies at 77. *New York Times* 17 January. Available at: www.nytimes.com/2016/01/18/books/peggy-anderson-chronicler-of-the-nursing-profession-dies-at-77.html.

Sasso L, Bagnasco A, Zanini M, Catania G, Aleo G, Santullo A, Spandonaro F, Icardi G, Watson R and Sermeus W (2017) The general results of the RN4CAST survey in Italy *Journal of Advanced Nursing* 73(9): 2028–2030.

Schulze B (2007) Stigma and mental health professionals: A review of the evidence on an intricate relationship *International Review of Psychiatry* 19 (2): 137–155.

Scorsese M (dir) (2010) *Shutter Island.* Film Hollywood: Paramount.

Sharp S, McAllister M and Broadbent M (2017) The tension between person centred and task focused care in an acute surgical setting: a critical ethnography *Collegian* 25: 11–18.

Skyman E, Sjöström H and Hellström L (2010) Patients' experiences of being infected with MRSA at a hospital and subsequently source isolated *Scandinavian Journal of Caring Sciences* 24 (1): 101–107.

Stanley D (2008) Celluloid angels: A research study of nurses in feature films 1900–2007 *Journal of Advanced Nursing* 64(1): 84–95.

Stanley D (2012) Celluloid devils: A research study of male nurses in feature films *Journal of Advanced Nursing* 68(11): 2526–2537.

Sullivan E (2002) Nursing and feminism: An uneasy alliance *Journal of Professional Nursing* 18(4): 183–184.

Templeton S (2004) Too clever to care for you. *The Sunday Times* 25 April. Available at: www.thetimes.co.uk/article/nurses-are-too-clever-to-care-for-you-275fdcfj658

Thomas G (dir) (1959) *Carry on Nurse.* Film. Buckinghamshire: Beaconsfield Productions.

Thomas G (dir) (1967) *Carry on Doctor.* Film. Buckinghamshire: Beaconsfield Productions.

Trinkoff A, Geiger-Brown J, Brady B, Lipscomb J and Muntaner C (2006) How long and how much are nurses now working? Too long, too much, and without enough rest between shifts, a study finds *The American Journal of Nursing* 106(4): 60–71.

Twyker T, Wachowski L and Wachowski L (dir) (2012). *Cloud Atlas.* Hollywood: Warner Brothers.

Watson R (creator) (1976–1983) *The Young Doctors.* Television series. Sydney: Reg Grundy Productions.

Werker A (dir) (1946) *Shock.* Film. Hollywood: 20th Century Fox.

7   Murdering nurses

Introduction

The German film *Fog in August* (Wessel, 2016) opens with the following scene:

> A pale young boy, his head shaven and wearing rags, is physically assessed by
> a doctor who seems kind and attentive. The doctor notices cuts and bruises
> on Ernst's small frame – the remnants of beatings he received in the boy's
> home from which he has been transferred. Ernst is the child of a Yenish
> family, one of the so-called "Gypsy" races, which included the Roma and
> Sinti people, and who today would be named "Travellers" (Murphy, 2017).
> As his family was stigmatised, and unable to find a permanent address, Ernst
> was classified as homeless. The doctor allocates him to farm work and directs
> the Head Orderly to take care of him. He also assures the child that he will
> not be beaten, and adds that there is no schooling available.

So begins Ernst's experience of life in a mental institution in Nazi Germany.
The film continues to show Ernst following an orderly out into the wards.
He is frightened by what he sees around him: physically and intellectually disabled children call for food and attention; adult mental patients scream and
struggle against the application of leather restraints. There are few staff and no
words of comfort for any of the patients who are largely left to fend for
themselves. In this institution, inmates do not survive long. The ostensibly
humane Medical Director has drawn up a list of young patients that the
nurses must prepare for transfer the following evening. An ominous grey bus,
its windows shrouded in paper, waits at the hospital entrance. Despite the terrible conditions of the institution, the children prefer to remain there than to
board that bus, suggesting its destination must be dire. The nurses, who are
Catholic nuns, comply with the order, but also attempt to make the passage
of the frightened children less threatening by leading them in a farewell song:
"Let me sing your sufferings. My compassion is my offering". The song's
words reveal that, while the children are being led to their deaths, the only
strategy the nurses have available to them is to show a little humanity.

Fog in August is an important film because it shines light on a largely hidden topic – nurses' involvement in systematic mass murder during the Nazi period. While, as the previous chapter profiles, the monstrous behaviour of evil nurses is a popular device in horror films, such appalling behaviour also occurs in real life but rarely attracts the sustained notice of figures such as Nurse Ratched from *One Flew Over the Cuckoo's Nest* (Forman, 1975; Kesey, 1962) and Annie Wilkes from *Misery* (King, 1987; Reiner, 1990). Because of this, its representation in a more realistic form in a fictional film based on actual events and individuals such as *Fog in August* can assist in the wider recognition that nurses have the knowledge, skills and means to kill. It is a disturbing fact that, alongside the narrative of nursing as dedicated, selfless and aimed at helping and benefiting the patient, there is a powerful thread of crime and corruption, including murder, running though nursing's history and contemporary practice. This is a major reason why establishing and monitoring standards, ethics and regulations in health care is so important.

Jung (1917) hypothesised that the shadow side of the self lies at the edge of the conscious and unconscious psyche and is a part of the natural order of each individual. This is the dark, unlived and suppressed side of the human self that contains the repressed memories, and primitive, negative and socially disparaged emotions and impulses. Rather than seeing this shadow side as a "problem" to be "solved", it is, instead, a mystery to be recognised and then confronted. Exploring this hidden shadow side also has the power to connect individuals to the depths of their imaginations and potential. Rather than acknowledge systemic or institutional faults and failings, many nurses push less than exemplary nursing practices and behaviours into the shadows; meaning that these shortcomings are duly avoided, hidden and unprocessed (Gray, 2009). Thinking of the nursing profession as a corpus with a collective unconscious, its shadow can be identified as that which has been, and is (and therefore remains) denied, hidden and unaddressed. Nurses' actions during the Holocaust is one such shadow.

Nursing's darkest hour

The scene from the film *Fog in August* at the beginning of this chapter alludes to the German Nazi policies that enacted a series of the most notorious acts of genocide in modern history. Over six million Jewish people and three million others were systematically murdered in what was an explicit Nazi policy aiming to rid Germany of people deemed to be inferior and a burden on the nation (Harran et al., 2000). While the incarceration, starvation and murder of Jewish and other people in concentration camps is widely acknowledged, Supremacism also saw the forced sterilisation of over 300,000 Germans who were considered to be carriers of hereditary diseases that would contaminate the nation's aspiration to racial purity (Gittelman, 2006). These beliefs also prompted the development of programs of selective breeding and the forced adoption of Aryan-looking children from invaded countries (Mouton, 2007).

An undoubtedly shameful but inescapable fact is that nurses – many of them highly qualified and professionally affiliated – played a key role in facilitating these atrocities (Benedict and Shields, 2014).

In the next scene from *Fog in August*, set in the hospital ward of the mental institution, frail and helpless children wait silently and resignedly to be fed. Amelie is dark haired and tiny. Anywhere between six to twelve years of age, Amelie refuses to eat and is wasting away. Next to her, a toddler with Down Syndrome smiles at her, innocently oblivious to the growing malevolence around them. Amelie stirs when Ernst enters the ward. Garrulous and naïvely optimistic, viewers learn that he has been transferred from the boy's home for being "unmanageable". As one of the stronger boys, he is still quick enough to evade the warders, and his help is grudgingly accepted by the overworked staff. Sitting at Amelie's bedside, he gently coaxes her into swallowing a few mouthfuls of porridge. All is quiet until a nurse enters the room, holding a glass of medicine on a tray. Dressed pristinely in white – a stark contrast to the dishevelled rags of the children – she stares ominously at Ernst, clear that her intentions have been foiled by his presence. She must try a different tack and gain his compliance.

> Nurse Kiefer smiles ingratiatingly, gently strokes his face and says, "Ernst, it is so sweet of you to help us. Will you let me sit down?"
> Ernst knows that he cannot object.
> Nurse Kiefer continues: "Hello, Amelie. Look what I've got you. Raspberry juice! Do you want it?"
> "What's it for?" Ernst asks suspiciously, for no one in German institutions has been able to secure such a delicacy since the war began.
> Nurse Kiefer ignores him and says to Amelie: "Only for you. Come on, open your mouth."
> "She doesn't want it!", Ernst protests protectively.
> Nurse Kiefer, momentarily losing her gentility, snaps back, "She has to! The Director ordered it!"
> Turning, the nurse says encouragingly but firmly, "Be a good girl now, Amelie. Drink your juice".
> Amelie resists weakly, but Nurse Kiefer persists. "Amelie, open your mouth. Amelie . . . ".
> Ernst reacts quickly, "I can do it!", for it is true that only Ernst is successful in cajoling Amelie into feeding.
> Nurse Kiefer gives the cup to him and Ernst approaches Amelie as the nurse watches.
> Just then, the ward sister and nun, Sister Sophia, enters the room. The sudden interruption provides Ernst with an opportunity to thwart Nurse Kiefer's deadly intent. He drops the cup and cries, "Oh Sorry! I didn't mean to do that".
> Ernst's courage has saved the little girl, for the moment at least.

This chilling scene alludes to the poisoning of children that was carried out by nurses in a number of German hospitals at the time the film is set.

Following a humiliating defeat in the First World War, the German nation set about reassembling its strength and prosperity. Increasingly, Germans were told, and came to believe, that they had a duty to their people collectively – the nation – and that this duty transcended individualism and personal desires and goals. This idea of duty, which was widely promulgated in propaganda including in popular cultural forms (Benedict, 2003), included: working hard; having large families; being fit and healthy by eating well, avoiding alcohol and cigarettes and engaging in regular outdoor exercise; attending State events; and, volunteering labour to the State (Proctor, 1996). Hitler encouraged women to become nurses, decreeing that, in doing so, they could perform the role of ultimate "mother" for Germany. In this role, although skilled from their professional training, nurses would also follow the "good nurse" trope and be constantly available, ever-nurturing selfless carers. Under the Nazi ideology, German nurses were encouraged to research and publish on health and wellbeing, professional standards were developed, and the whole profession enjoyed a significant elevation in their social status (Steppe, 1992).

National commitment to strengthening the nation by creating a pure German race took hold and what was described as a "positive eugenics" programme was initiated. In Germany, women were awarded medals for having large numbers of children, while birth statistics were gathered and all defective births reported and recorded (Holmes, McAllister and Crowther, 2016). Germany was not alone in this interest. The "science" of eugenics was being studied and enacted in Europe and the US at the end of the late nineteenth century (Benedict, 2014). Its basic theory draws from Social Darwinism – the survival of the fittest – which was distorted to assert that the human race could (and should) advance through the destruction of its weakest members. While this approach to population was popular all over the world in the early part of the twentieth century, eugenics had a dark side. Countless numbers of people with intellectual or mental problems were forcibly institutionalised and sterilised because there was a widespread belief that they were inferior and would bring down the collective health of the population (Currell and Cogdell, 2006). This theory was applied rigidly under National Socialism in Germany and communicated through widespread propaganda programmes (Benedict, 2003). Hitler's rise to power in 1933 began the process of implementation of policies designed to incorporate eugenic practices under the guise of "euthanasia" (Benedict and Chelouche, 2008). Among the first victims of this policy were children with impairments or disabilities.

In another powerful scene from *Fog in August*, the hospital's Medical Director calls Sister Sophia and Head Orderly Hechtle to his office to announce that the T4 programme had officially been cancelled by the Fuhrer. Sister Sophia allows herself a moment of relief. Her religious belief in the sanctity of all life had meant that she was an unwilling accomplice to the crimes at work in the institution. She had been in a state of constant tension because she had been compelled by her superiors to do what she could to care for the inmates who she knew were going to be killed. She whispers a brief, "Thank God", and turns to return to her duties. But then the Director tells Hechtle that the procedure would continue, although in a changed format. The convoys of conspicuous grey buses that would leave the institution filled with children and return later that day, carrying only their luggage, had raised the suspicion and outrage of the villagers. Remarking sadly, "The people simply do not understand the wisdom of the policy yet", he explains that Berlin had decreed that the programme needed to continue locally, but unofficially. Staff were ordered to continue to select the weakest from the patient group, stop feeding them and administer barbiturates to induce respiratory depression and death. The Orderly asks a practical question, "Who will carry it out?", to which the Director responds: "Anyone willing to help release the sick from their misery will receive an extra thirty Reichsmarks".

The policy alluded to in this scene is the Nazi eugenics policy, known as the *Action T4 Program* (T4). T4 began in 1938 with an order from Hitler and was then communicated by Nazi officials to specific hospitals across the country. It represented a paradigm shift in Nazi politics, evolving from a nationalist policy aiming to strengthen the population through mass public health campaigns to a demonic agenda that sought to eradicate the weak and unwanted. This order decreed that doctors were to select and kill disabled children who met the criteria of being "unfit to live" – those deemed to be "hereditarily sick" or "incurably ill" – as well as people from non-Aryan racial backgrounds (Burleigh, 1994). The policy was euphemistically referred to as "euthanasia" – the literal meaning of which is "peaceful death" (Harris, 2001). To bolster the policy's legitimacy and garner support from health professionals, medical institutions were renamed and given grand titles such as "Reich Committee Institute" and the nurses and doctors who worked within them were, as the film suggests, given higher pay and praised for being good Nazi citizens and contributing to a strengthening nation (Holmes, McAllister and Crowther, 2016).

The T4 program began by killing newborns diagnosed with illnesses such as microcephaly, cerebral palsy and any malformations of the limbs (Lifton, 1986). Midwives were required to report cases to doctors, who were, in turn, required to notify the ministry. By 1940, the selection criteria became looser and included children up to the age of four years of age, and then older children, adults with illnesses and those considered racially impure. Notions of what constituted "illness" and "incurability" have since evolved but, at that time, people who were homosexuals, drug dependent, prostitutes, from Slavic countries, Poles and Jews fell within the criteria of "unfit for life" and were victims of this policy of extermination (Lifton, 1986). The criteria also included people with mental illnesses, the elderly and ailing soldiers (Fuller-Torrey and Yolken, 2010). Most killed under this programme did not have incurable diseases, nor were their deaths peaceful. Thus, even at the time when it was being instituted and carried out, the T4 policy could not be described as euthanasia. It was murder and genocide, sanitised under the guise of pseudo-science policy. In today's terms – which defines euthanasia as the legal act of intentionally ending a life to relieve pain and suffering, and especially that of a person or an animal which is terminally ill or fatally injured (Harris, 2001) – this Nazi T4 practice would not be considered euthanasia, because the patients were not dying, did not give consent, and nor were they necessarily suffering from their disease. What occurred was that these "patients" were medically murdered by health professionals. Nurses and nursing orderlies were directed to carry out the killing. Most of the hospitals in which these murders occurred were church-run and, therefore, ostensibly operating under the Christian ethos that honoured the sanctity of all life. However, under the Nazi ideology, health care managers and workers, including nurses, underwent a significant shift in values. In addition to being involved in the facilitation of health and wellbeing which underpinned the tenets of professional health care, these individuals also became involved in the facilitation of death – a monumental shift in professional values, and one that even now is difficult to understand and accept. So difficult indeed, that this is only just emerging as a topic of public discussion now, with films such as *Fog in August* bringing the topic into public view.

This is despite historical research such as that carried out by Steppe more than twenty-five years ago, which interviewed some of the participating nurses. Steppe's important research found that a significant portion of German nurses accepted this Nazi reinterpretation of professional nursing ethics in the assumption that, through their obedience to directives, they were doing good (Steppe, 1992). The need to comply with the T4 policy was reinforced through the widespread Nazi propaganda programme that continually stated, and reinforced, the belief that the German Aryan people were superior to all others (Burleigh and Wippermann, 1991). Both anti-Jewish, and anti-disability, propaganda were ubiquitous. Stories appeared in newspapers, on the radio, posted on buses and in other public locations, featured in films and other programming in cinemas, and in art and children's books, that people who were a burden on society were evil, bestial, rat-like and contaminating German purity from within. This rhetoric was also repeated in nursing training manuals (Burleigh, 1994), and prompted the kind of distorted thinking known as dehumanisation.

The depiction of certain groups of people as inferior, dangerous and a financial drain on society made it easier for nurses and others to regard such patients as not fully human and believe that, as such, they could – and should – be eliminated for the good of the nation. Many nurses and doctors succumbed to these ideas of dehumanisation and lost all empathy for those supposedly in their care. As a result, the individual rights of members of these groups ceased to exist. These patients were killed by a range of means, either through starvation, lethal injection, drug overdoses or asphyxiation using carbon monoxide and, later, cyanide gas delivered in buses and specially constructed rooms made to look like showers in hospital basements (Heberer, 2008). Deliberate starvation involved purposefully feeding meals containing inadequate nutrition to sustain life, as is portrayed in *Fog in August*.

This excerpt from the actual trial that took place to prosecute the nurses working at one of the hospitals – Hadamar, near Limburg in the State of Hesse – describes the killing routine which was operationalised in order for the hospital to become a "euthanasia centre":

> On June 5 or 6, 1944, 75 laborers arrived from Hersfeld including 14 women and 2 children. As chief female nurse, Huber ordered the female nurses under her to prepare rooms for the new arrivals. They moved German patients to other rooms, ensured that the beds had fresh linens, and put the arriving patients to bed. Two male nurses, Ruoff and Willig, told the patients that they were being treated for communicable diseases and gave them the lethal oral medications and injections. Within 2 hours of arrival on the wards, the patients were dead. All were buried in mass graves. The sanitarium secretary, Judith Thomas, prepared death certificates. The institution's physician, Alolf Wahlmann, filled in the cause of death as lung disease and signed each certificate. He did not examine the patients before or after their deaths. Office worker Adolf Merkle falsified the dates of death by as much as a month. Over the next 10 months, the process was repeated countless times.
>
> (Lagerwey, 1999, p. 761)

This evidence is revealing. Nurses systematically and efficiently lied to, and killed, large numbers of people, and then hid and falsified their means of death. In *Fog in August*, clinicians were also rewarded for their efforts with financial bonuses. What is so troubling, and chilling, is how the process – in both Germany and the film – mimicked procedures of proper nursing care. Following the matron's directions earlier, for instance, the nurses provide clean freshly made beds, utilise seeming state-of-the-art medical technology in the form of injections and medicines, and complete the proper documentation such as formal death certificates.

While there must have been nurses and doctors who refused to comply with these orders, there is no evidence from the Holocaust Studies or other literature that any nurse or doctor lost their job or was otherwise severely punished for non-participation and thus, it must be assumed that many of these health care professionals engaged willingly in the systematic process of selecting and killing patients, and then covered up these crimes using medical and administrative practices and protocols (Benedict and Shields, 2014; Foth, 2013). This atrocious part of nursing's history thus reveals how powerfully prevailing ideology can influence nursing actions, and override previously-developed professional values. Nurses working in National Socialist Germany were overwhelmingly compliant with the policies that sanctioned widespread killing, in place of caring and, even when the atrocity was over, many nurses denied their wrongdoing, protesting that they were as caring as well as possible for the poor patients, whose lives had become intolerable (Benedict, 2003). They were, they attested, putting people out of their misery. Steppe contends that the collective error that nurses made during this time was to believe that they were unaffected by the social, political and other changes taking place around them. This "apolitical professional consciousness" (Steppe, 1992, p. 744) made it possible for the profession to be subsumed by the larger political system and its goals. But, Steppe argues, nursing is socio-cultural and, as such, never takes place in a value-free, neutral context. And, she contends, nursing is always a socially significant force, that can be used for good or evil.

Where ethical principles include provision of autonomy, justice, beneficence and non-maleficence, these clinicians displayed the opposite. They defended their actions by saying to themselves and others that they were acting out of mercy – that to kill a disabled child or adult was to relieve them of prolonged suffering. Their actions, however, breached all notions of trust and patient autonomy and resulted in unnecessary suffering and brutal deaths.

Moreover, to suggest that the phenomenon of nurses killing instead of caring for people was an aberration brought on by the despotic policies of Nazi Germany, and the evils of the regime – and is, therefore, unlikely ever to occur again – is naïve. Nurses have killed patients on many other occasions and in a wide range of contexts. As shown so vividly in *Fog in August,* nurses have access to the means and the power to make decisions about who lives and dies, as well as when, and how, they die.

Angels of death

A number of more contemporary nurses have been found guilty of what is termed "medical murder". Dubbed "Angels of Death" (Vronsky, 2004, and others), these nurses are anything but angelic. This Angel of Death metaphor is, moreover, a sanitised description of health care workers who carry out killings, sometimes in the name of mercy or for other reasons. Yet, the moniker, "Angel of Death", infers only that death occurred, not that it was caused by an act of murder and, further, that – due to the presence of a heavenly being – the patient has been mercifully killed. A more apt description, however, is to describe the act as "medical murder", for the behaviour is predatory and obscene (Hickey, 2010) and occurs in the medical setting, perpetrated by medical workers, including nurses. Yardley and Wilson define the health care serial killer as "a doctor or a nurse, sometimes working within a hospital, the community, a nursing home or simply a healthcare professional using their medical skills to murder" (2016, p 40). Today, nurses deliberately killing patients remains a rare phenomenon. Approximately ninety such murderers have been identified and reported in the academic literature between 1970 and 2006

(Yardley and Wilson, 2016). This does not, however, include some known terrible offenders such as the Australian nurses Roger Dean and Pamela Rose Jenkin, and others who had not then been detected at the time of writing. Although these murdering nurses are relatively rare, they are terrifying because there is evidence that they may be attracted to health care as a means to access victims and because the trust afforded to health care workers gives such killers a means to remain undetected for some time.

When the actions of contemporary murderous nurses become known, these cases are widely represented in the popular media, in reports by journalists, documentaries, biographies and films "based on a true story" as well as true crime books and podcasts. Podcasts that retell the stories of, and/or offer an analysis of, actual crimes are attracting large and committed audiences (Tinker, 2018). Most of these popular productions, whether in print, on screen or online, make, and underscore, the same point that nurses have the knowledge, skill and means to kill. They also frequently reveal the flaws in health service provision, regulation and governance that allow these criminals to flourish before they are caught.

Yardley and Wilson (2016) warn that common features of such killers are that they are accomplished con artists, often craving attention and displaying what has been described as a "hero-complex". Such nurses use their authority to target vulnerable groups such as sick children or the elderly. While the patient may be sick, they are not usually terminally ill, and known motivations for their acts of murder include wanting to rid themselves of demanding patients, free up beds or gain attention (Askill and Sharpe, 2014). Nurses who said they killed out of pity and to end patients' suffering include Pamela Rose Jenkin, Stephen Letter and the so-called Lainz Angels of Death; while nurses who portrayed pathological attention-seeking or flagrant abuse of power and callous disregard for life include Beverly Allitt, Richard Angelo, Joseph Dewey Akin, Charles Cullen, Benjamin Geen and Genene Jones. Most often, these are nowhere near what might constitute "merciful deaths". Field describes these individuals' profiles as extremely diverse, and as broad as the hiring profile of nursing itself:

> Some are clearly extremely intelligent; others are not. Some are young, some are older, some are male, some are female, some are gay, some are straight, some are senior nurses, some are mere assistants, but all are able to murder patients.
>
> (2007, p. 316)

A recent example is that of American nurse Charles Cullen, whose story is told in a popular true crime biography, the ironically titled *The Good Nurse: A True Story of Medicine Madness and Murder* by Charles Graeber (2014), a *New York Times* bestseller. Cullen was arrested in 2003 after a police investigation found him the most likely perpetrator of the murder of five patients and implicated in the deaths of almost three hundred. Cullen later confessed to killing forty patients in nine hospitals and a nursing home over a sixteen-year period (Yorker et al., 2006). If Cullen did murder all those that he is suspected of killing, it would make him one of the most prolific serial killers of all time (Graeber, 2014). Ironically, however, Cullen was not described as a monster by his colleagues, who believed him a good, or even an excellent, nurse. To earn this title as a man in nursing, it is plausible to suggest that he must have displayed exceptional nursing virtues. Descriptions from *The Good Nurse* dispel the myth that such killers are easy to identify:

> Nurse Cullen appeared to be an ideal hire. His attendance was perfect, his uniform pristine. He had experience in intensive care, critical care, cardiac care, ventilation, and burns. He medicated the living, was the first code responder when machines screamed over the dying, and exhibited origami-like artistry when plastic-wrapping the dead.
>
> (p. 4)

He was, moreover, an extremely willing worker:

> He had no scheduling conflicts, didn't seem to attend movies or watch sports, and was willing, even eager, to work nights, weekends, and holidays . . . a last-second sick call or an unexpected patient transfer could have him dressed and on the highway before the commercial break. His fellow nurses considered him a gift from the scheduling gods, a hire almost too good to be true.
>
> (p. 4)

In Graeber's narrative, Cullen is also described as efficient, seemingly ever-attentive to patients and skilled with medical technology. His actions, however, are clearly the opposite of good nursing – and this is why Cullen was so dangerous. In common with other serial killers (Simpson, 2017), Cullen demonstrated a lack, or a diffuseness, of identity. On one hand, he came across at times as innocuous and inoffensive, while on the other, he also had an alter-ego that coldly, efficiently and randomly injected bolus doses of dangerous drugs into IV bags that could then be administered to any patient on the ward, relatively untraceably. Ultimately, although he seemed to have all the qualities that made a good nurse, he had none of what would have made him a good person.

Over Cullen's fourteen-year nursing career, he worked in a large number of health services, all of which failed to report suspicious incidents and an increased rate of death for fear that such actions might trigger lawsuits or other legal ramifications (Perez-Pena, Kocieniewski and George, 2004). In the Somerset Medical Centre case, for example, when Cullen was suspected of both a murder and an attempted murder (Graeber, 2014, p. 173), the hospital's lawyers stressed the risk to the hospital's reputation and "requested that all interviews be conducted within the hospital, in the presence of [their] Risk Manager" (p. 176). In one case, when enquiries were made, his personnel file had mysteriously disappeared and, in another, his presence at the hospital was completely deleted from the system.

Such systemic defensiveness and corruption is not unique to Cullen's case. When Genene Jones was suspected of being responsible for the deaths of up to sixty babies and children in her care, hospital staff are reported to have refused to cooperate with the investigation for fear of litigation from past or present patients (Elkind, 1989). After she was convicted for causing one death, hospitals reportedly destroyed their records with the express purpose of avoiding such litigation. Jones' story has featured in a number of popular book-length and screen true crime biographies and exposés (Moore and Reed, 1988; Elkind, 1989; Colla, 1991; Meyers, 2002) as well as episodes in television and podcast series on murderers and women criminals. In the case of Richard Angelo, who deliberately injected paralysing drugs into as many as thirty patients in order to "rescue" them and then be praised for doing so, the quality assurance standards of the hospital were reportedly so poor that it would have been impossible to detect any nurse misadministering medications, let alone deliberately poisoning patients (Evening News, 1987). The Lainz Killers case was similar. In the 1980s in Vienna, four female Austrian nursing assistants collaborated to kill feeble elderly patients, using overdoses of morphine or by holding them down in bed and filling their mouths with water, holding their noses until they breathed in and drowned. This quartet are alleged to have killed up to a hundred patients in this way. Again, the hospital was strongly criticised for refusing to cooperate with the investigation, instead raising "a wall of silence" (Anon., 1989, p. A10).

Although these stories are enshrined in the relevant legal cases, when they feature in popular culture retellings, the public can really come to understand the situations, people and systemic failures involved. The cases above, for instance, all reveal that hospital corruption is also culpable in these dire scenarios. Many deaths could have been avoided, and lives saved, had the hospital managers been more motivated by their higher duty to patient safety, and more willing to allow their flawed systems be open to scrutiny. Systemic failures lie at the centre of these human tragedies. Accessible representations in popular culture can distill these complex descriptions and sometimes confusing sequences of events into powerful narratives that compel our attention and endure in popular memory (Lipsitz, 1990; Middleweek, 2017).

The Beverley Allitt case is a clear example of this. Allitt was an English nurse who had experienced abuse in her own childhood and had a history of hospitalisations for non-existent illnesses. Reportedly long wanting to become a paediatric nurse, Allitt volunteered as a babysitter, then found work in a small English village hospital as an enrolled nurse. There she murdered at least four children and attempted to kill at least five others over a two-month period in 1991. The methods she used included suffocation, and administering overdoses of insulin and air-filled injections. At the same time, she would befriend her ailing patients' parents, even becoming godmother to one of her victims. This crime has attracted multiple retellings in popular culture. Apart from widespread newspaper articles, these narratives include a number of true crime books (Askill and Sharpe, 2014; Davies, 1993; Parris, 2017) and a movie-length BBC dramatisation of the story titled *Angel of Death* (Proctor, 2005). Allitt's story was also retold over the next two decades in episodes of true crime series including *Crimes That Shook Great Britain* (2008–current) (Le Han, 2008), *Born To Kill?* (2005–current) (Williams, 2012), *Evil Up Close* (-2012–14) (Murray, 2012) and *Nurses Who Kill* (Jury, 2016). Allitt's story also features in recent true crime podcast series including *Once Upon and Crime* (Ludlow, 2017) and *True Crime Brewery* ("Jill and Dick", 2017). In their representation of Allitt, her actions and their ramifications, these narratives in the popular media all relate a number features in common: the horrendous details of the crimes Allitt committed; suggestions that Allitt became a nurse in order to kill; her active befriending of the victims' families; and, how warning signs about her behaviour were "overlooked" or ignored (Foster, 1994). In these re-tellings of her crimes, all these elements – from those personal to Allitt, to flaws in the health care system – are presented as having contributed to Allitt's crimes.

It is a paradox that these aspects of evil and purposeful failure in health care are represented in forensic detail in popular culture and, yet, nursing scholarship offers little theorising about nursing's involvement in this macabre constellation (Holmes, McAllister and Crowther, 2016). Consequently, many nursing students and practicing nurses are unaware of, and certainly not fully briefed about, the events and crimes discussed in this chapter. If there was more widespread awareness and open discussions of such situations and their tragic outcomes, perhaps more nurses would feel empowered to take action against the growing incidence of preventable deaths occurring in nursing homes (Ibrahim et al., 2017), address systemic causes of neglectful care (Bogner, 2018), and conscientiously object to harmful policies and practices (Vogus, Sutcliffe and Weick, 2010).

Conclusion

Although neither medicine in general, nor the nursing profession in particular, seems willing or currently equipped to consider evil behaviour and its ramification in detail, popular culture provides a means to introduce this topic into general discourse and, moreover, keep these crimes in the public eye. The representations of murdering nurses in popular culture also provides a range of suggestions as to why these human and systemic failures may have occurred. In the case of the nurses in Nazi Germany who participated in the medicalised murders of vulnerable children and adults, *Fog in August* powerfully reveals how nurses were caught up in acts of killing, neglect and corrupt practices and the motivations, justifications and morality involved. These nurses typically dehumanised their patients. They demonstrated little compassion or care, and became so involved in this obscene behaviour that they even desired, and enabled, its continuance after the orders regarding its perpetration had ceased. While it is tempting, and comforting, to minimise the significance of these nurses' acts with such claims as "nurses were not as educated or empowered then as they are now" or "nurses were being told what to do and they were only following orders" looking to Jung's acknowledgement of the shadow can provide a deeper and more persuasive route to understanding how this could have occurred. Jung explains that the first step to understanding evil is through acknowledging that we all have potential to do bad things. Individuals must come to understand both "how much good" they can do and "what crimes [they are] . . . capable of" (1963, p. 330). In therapy, individuals taking a Jungian approach engage in "shadow work", where attempts are made to bring unconscious processes to the surface of the conscious mind to achieve wholeness (Zweig and Wolf, 1997). This quest for wholeness can only be achieved when this shadow is acknowledged and faced, and this recognition assimilated into one's sense of identity. For a community such as nursing, collective "shadow work" involves facing past evils, and taking moral, political and spiritual responsibility for dark actions and darker days. As Tarrant proposes, "the courage with which we bear our darkness frees others from having to carry it for us" (1998, p. 170).

These and other cases of contemporary and historical murdering nurses also build the strongest case that nurses cannot be bystanders when the law, human rights or ethics are being infringed or when corrupt policies are being enacted. Nurses have a duty to speak out when harm occurs to patients or when one social group is treated inequitably in the health care system. Whatever the political or social atmosphere, however strong the peer pressure, nurses must remain alert to signs of inhumanity. In doing so, they must call into question the principles that are believed to underpin the traditional trope of the good nurse, and replace these with professional competence, professionalism and self-consciousness which is empowered to challenge any wrong doing. Not least, as Steppe implores, nurses have a moral obligation to the millions of victims of National Socialism to ensure that nursing actions during that time are not forgotten. As she proposes, speaking about the nursing profession, "by taking responsibility for this part of our history, we can become more sensitive for the future, with eyes and ears open for all social injustice" (p. 744).

References

Anonymous (1989) Death angels revive memories of Nazi times. *The Spokesman-Review/Spokane Chronicle* 16 April: A10.

Askill J and Sharpe M (2014) *Angel of Death: Killer Nurse Beverly Allitt.* London: Michael O'Mara Books.

Benedict S (2003) Killing while caring: The nurses of Hadamar. *Issues in Mental Health Nursing* 24: 59–79.

Benedict S (2014) Fertile ground for murder. In Benedict S and Shields L (eds) *Nurses and Midwives in Nazi Germany: The "Euthanasia Programs".* New York: Routledge, 13–26.

Benedict S and Chelouche T (2008) Meseritz-Obrawalde: A 'wild euthanasia' hospital of Nazi Germany. *History of Psychiatry* 19(1): 68–76.

Benedict S and Shields L (2014) *Nurses and Midwives in Nazi Germany: The "euthanasia Programs".* New York: Routledge.

Bogner M (ed) (2018) *Human Error in Medicine.* New Jersey: Lawrence Erlbaum Press.

Burleigh M (1994) *Death and Deliverance.* Cambridge: Cambridge University Press.

Burleigh M and Wippermann W (1991) *The Racial State: Germany 1933–1945.* Cambridge: Cambridge University Press.

Colla R dir (1991) Deadly medicine. *Television.* New York: NBC.

Currell S and Cogdell C (2006) *Popular Eugenics: National Efficiency and American Mass Culture in the 1930s.* Athens, OH: Ohio University Press.

Davies N (1993) *Murder on Ward Four: The Story of Bev Allitt and the Most Terrifying Crime since the Moors Murders.* London: Chatto and Windus.

Elkind P (1989) *The Death Shift: The True Story of Nurse Genene Jones and the Texas Baby Murders.* New York: Viking.

The Evening News (1987) State cites "Angel of Death" hospital for shortcomings. *The Evening News* 18 December.

Forman M dir (1975) One Flew Over the Cuckoo's Nest. *Film.* Hollywood: Fantasy Films.

Foster J (1994) Warning signs about Allitt "overlooked". *The Independent.* 2 February. Available at: www.independent.co.uk/news/uk/warning-signs-about-allitt-overlooked-1391435.html.

Foth T (2013) Understanding "caring" through biopolitics: The case of nurses under the Nazi regime. *Nursing Philosophy* 14: 284–294.

Fuller-Torrey E and Yolken R (2010) Psychiatric genocide: Nazi attempts to eradicate schizophrenia. *Schizophrenia Bulletin* 36(1): 26–32.

Gittelman M (2006) The Holocaust, racism, mental illness: Editor's introduction. *International Journal of Mental Health* 35(3): 5–16.

Graeber C (2014) *The Good Nurse: A True Story of Medicine, Madness and Murder.* New York: Hachette Book Group.

Gray B (2009) The emotional labour of nursing: Defining and managing emotions in nursing work. *Nurse Education Today* 29(2): 168–175.

Harran M, Kuntz D, Lemons R, Michael R, Pickus K and Roth J (2000) *The Holocaust Chronicle.* San Diego: Publications International.

Harris N (2001) The euthanasia debate. *Journal of the Royal Army Medical Corps* 147(3): 367–370.

Heberer P (2008) Early postwar justice in the American zone: The 'Hadamar murder factory' trial. In Heberer P and Matthäus J (eds) *Atrocities on Trial: Historical Perspectives on the Politics of Prosecuting War Crimes.* Lincoln: University of Nebraska Press, 25–47.

Hickey E (2010) *Serial Murderers and Their Victims. 5th ed.* Belmont: Wadsworth.

Holmes C, McAllister M and Crowther A (2016) Nurses writing about psychiatric nurses' involvement in killings during the Nazi era: A preliminary discourse analysis. *Health and History Journal* 18(2): 63–84.

Ibrahim J, Bugeja L, Willoughby M, Bevan M, Kipsaina C, Young C, Pham T and Ranson D (2017) Premature deaths of nursing home residents: An epidemiological analysis. *The Medical Journal of Australia* 206(10): 442–447.

Jill and Dick (2017) No mercy: The victims of killer nurse Beverley Allitt. Podcast. *True Crime Brewery*. Available at: https://tiegrabber.com/podcasts/no-mercy-the-victims-of-killer-nurse-beverly-allitt/.

Jung C (1917) *On the Psychology of the Unconscious. Collected Works of C.G. Jung, Vol. 7.* Princeton: Princeton University Press.

Jung C (1963) *Memories, Dreams, Reflections.* London: Vintage.

Jury C dir. (2016) Beverely Allitt. *Nurses Who Kill* episode 1, series 1. Television series. Stratford upon Avon: Firstlook TV.

Kesey K (1962) *One Flew Over The Cuckoo's Nest.* London: Pan Books.

King S (1987) *Misery.* New York: Hodder and Stoughton.

King W (1984) Five given injections quit breathing, doctor says in nurse's trial. *The New York Times*, 6 February.

Lagerwey M (1999) Nursing ethics at Hadamar. *Qualitative Health Research* 9(6): 759–772.

Le Han M dir (2008) Beverley allitt. *Crimes That Shook Britain* season 1, episode 1. Television series. UK: A+E networks.

Lifton R (1986) German doctors and the final solution. *The New York Times Magazine* 21 September. Available at: www.nytimes.com/1986/09/21/magazine/german-doctors-and-the-final-solution.html.

Lipsitz G (1990) *Time Passages: Collective Memory and American Popular Culture.* Minneapolis: University of Minnesota Press.

Ludlow E (2017) Sick and murdered: Beverley Allitt. Podcast. *Once Upon a Crime* episode 55. Available at: www.onceuponacrime.libsyn.com.

Meyers J (dir) (2002) *Mass Murder.* Video. imdb.com.

Middleweek B (2017) Dingo media?: The persistence of the "trial by media" frame in popular, media, and academic evaluations of the Azaria Chamberlain case. *Feminist Media Studies* 17(3): 392–411.

Moore K and Reed D (1988) *Deadly Medicine.* New York: St Martin's Press.

Mouton M (2007) *From Nurturing the Nation to Purifying the Volk: Weimar and Nazi Family Policy, 1918–1945.* Cambridge: Cambridge University Press.

Murphy D (2017) Ethnic minorities in Europe: The Yenish (Yeniche) people. *Traveller's Voice*. Available at: www.travellersvoice.ie/2017/07/25/ethnic-minorities-in-europe-the-yenish-yeniche-people.

Murray R (dir) (2012) The ward assassin: Beverly allitt. *Evil Up Close* episode 4, season 1. Television series. Stratford upon Avon: First Look TV.

Parris J (2017) *Killer Nurse Beverly Allitt.* Scotts Valley: CreateSpace Independent Publishing.

Perez-Pena R, Kocieniewski D and George J (2004) Death on the night shift: 16 years, dozens of bodies. Through gaps in system, nurse left trail of grief. *New York Times* 29 February. Available at: www.nytimes.com/2004/02/29/nyregion/death-night-shift-16-years-dozens-bodies-through-gaps-system-nurse-left-trail.html.

Proctor C (casting dir) (2005) *Angel of Death: The Beverly Allitt Story*. London: BBC.

Proctor R (1996) The anti-tobacco campaign of the Nazis: A little known aspect of public health in Germany, 1933–45. *British Medical Journal* 313(7070): 1450–1453.

Reiner R dir (1990) *Misery*. Film. Hollywood: Castlerock Entertainment.

Simpson P (2017) *The Serial Killer Files*. Sydney: Hachette Books.

Steppe H (1992) Nursing in Nazi Germany. *Western Journal of Nursing Research* 14(6): 744–753.

Tarrant J (1998) *The Light inside the Dark: Zen, Soul, and the Spiritual Life*. New York: Harper Collins.

Tinker R (2018) Guilty pleasure: A case study of true crime's resurgence in a binge consumption era. *Elon Journal of Undergraduate Research in Communications* 9(1): 95–107.

Vogus T, Sutcliffe K and Weick K (2010) Doing no harm: Enabling, enacting, and elaborating a culture of safety in health care. *The Academy of Management Perspectives* 24(4): 60–77.

Vronsky P (2004) *Serial Killers: The Method and Madness of Monsters*. London: Penguin.

Wessel K dir (2016) *Fog in August*. Film. Paris: Studio Canal.

Williams T dir (2012) Beverley Allitt. *Born To Kill?* Television series. London: Channel 5 Television.

Yardley E and Wilson D (2016) In Search of the 'Angels of death': Conceptualising the contemporary nurse healthcare serial killer. *Journal of Investigative Psychology and Offender Profiling* 13(1): 39–55.

Yorker B, Kizer K, Lampe P, Forrest A, Lannan J and Russell D (2006) Serial murder by healthcare professionals *Journal of Forensic Sciences* 51(6): 1362–1371.

Zweig C and Wolf S (1997) *Romancing the Shadow: Illuminating the Dark Side of the Soul*. New York: Ballantine Books.

8 Nurses and sick health care systems

Introduction

In previous chapters, numerous paradoxes that challenge nurses and shape nursing's identity have been discussed, including the expectation that nurses be highly educated and technically competent and yet they possess knowledge that is looked upon with suspicion or confusion. Another paradox is that nurses utilise many ways of knowing to inform clinical reasoning as well as compassionate care but sometimes even nurses are in a state of unknowing and uncertainty, particularly in the face of horrifying situations and the unexplainable. Nurses are one of the most highly trusted professions in society, yet sometimes that trust can be breached in the most grievous ways. Nurses are expected to prioritise caring values and yet have, at times, been a party to corruption, criminality and even genocide. Such inconsistencies create instability in identity for some nurses – leading some to question "Am I an important health professional or a servant to be directed"? or "Am I a change agent or a lowly pawn in the system"? – making them vulnerable to role dissatisfaction, disengagement, stress and burnout. One final irony important to discuss is that nurses, who occupy the greatest percentage of workers within the health workforce, are role models for health and yet sometimes cannot find a way through sick health care systems.

To fight for what is right

Within the first few moments of the BBC drama series *Trust Me* (2017), the scene is set regarding an inadequately resourced health care system that is falling inexorably into dysfunction. Cath Hardacre (played by Jodie Whittaker) is an experienced and caring RN managing busy NHS wards somewhere in Northern England. Over time, she has become frustrated with a series of damaging bureaucratic inactions: the hospital's failure to act over dangerously low standards of care, the lack of respect afforded to nurses, and the dearth of resources required for her role. An old woman is left to lie in sodden sheets and, while inexperienced interns fumble over the insertion of an IV, their patient goes into cardiac arrest. After doing her best to remedy these situations, including reporting the issues to the hospital's management, it is clear that the problems are too entrenched for Cath to resolve individually. Deciding to take action outsde the system, Cath then leaks confidential information on on these issues to an investigative journalist. He refuses to run the story unless Cath's identity is revealed. The questions for Cath are whether she will stand up and have the courage of her convictions and, in doing so, if she is prepared to expose herself and family in this way. This gripping premise builds on the real-life systemic failures of care in Stafford Hospital (Francis, 2013) in England, where up to 1,000 patients suffered and died because of widespread neglect. The whistleblower in this case, Helene Donnelly RN, was suspended for insisting on higher standards, persisting with her use of the internal complaint system and, finally, reporting the situation to the highest level of the NHS (Calkin, 2011).

It is a paradox that nurses can sometimes work within corrupt systems of care and reproduce the status quo, while others seek to change processes and system to improve them. For others, developments in nursing knowledge and advancements in practice do not necessarily, or directly, lead to satisfaction. This is also represented in popular culture, with the lead character in *Nurse Jackie*, for example, who is a highly skilled nurse, but neither her nursing work nor her nursing identity bring her happiness or financial stability. Furthermore, the ongoing educational reforms which have resulted in nurses becoming more knowledgeable and proficient in their work has not made a perceptible difference to the ways that hospitals are run. Frustration, burn-out, negligence, corruption and widespread awareness that systemic dysfunction is mightier than individual protest, still occurs.

This complex paradox underlies the clever writing of *Trust Me*. When the journalist explains that he must include the whistleblower's name for the story to run, Cath is placed in an untenable position. To see justice done, she risks losing her job and the meagre income she receives as the sole breadwinner for her family. Frustrated, she returns to the obsequious hospital board for one last appeal to their decency. Not only do they reject her request to investigate the cases more fully but coldly, and shockingly, they then turn the tables on her. They tell Cath that the board has received three complaints of bullying against her, and that she is to be suspended immediately pending a full investigation. Stunned and humiliated, but also desperate to find a way to earn an income, Cath resorts to impersonating an emergency department doctor. With this plot twist, the preliminary story of a fight for justice transforms into a crime thriller as Cath Hardacre, the extremely competent RN, becomes Ally Sutton, MD. Sutton is a friend and colleague of Cath's who despairs of the NHS's problems so much that she is leaving its service, and indeed, England, to become a farmer's wife in New Zealand. At (the real) Ally's farewell party, the partygoers – most of whom are nurses and doctors – raise a toast to the demise of the NHS. This indicates their deep dissatisfaction with their working lives, together with a pessimism that the situations caused by ongoing underfunding are ever likely to improve. As such, *Trust*

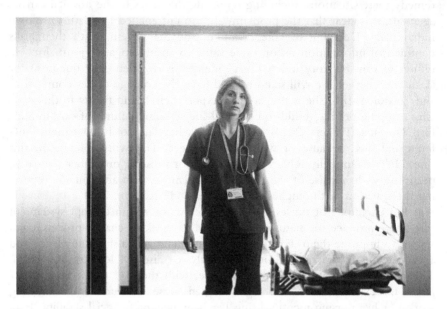

Figure 8.1 Cath Hardacre, RN a.k.a. Ally Sutton, MD – a victim or the product of a sick
health care system?

Me can be categorised as a dystopian view of modern health care; almost no
one who works in the system is either trusting or trustworthy. The unrelenting work-pressures, job shortages and lack of resources has led to
a generalised disillusionment and, as a result, a NHS workforce in crisis.

While the plot sounds far-fetched, the series writer Dan Sefton is also an
emergency doctor (Wallaston, 2017) who knows well that imposters do not
only work in health care but that they also create havoc (Gough, 1998; Evan,
1999), with recent cases exposed internationally (Murray et al., 2011; Poulsen,
2016). What makes the story of *Trust Me* both ambiguous and compelling is
how, while a serious manipulative criminal, the Cath/Ally character is also portrayed sympathetically. Although she is commiting a serious crime in impersonating a doctor and is barely competent, she studies hard and is more attentive
and kinder to the patients and the staff she works with than most of her peers
in the busy emergency department in which she finds work. Her motivation is
not cruelty or sadism, but family preservation. In a way, Cath maintains, and
displays, some of the traits of the good nurse – being compassionate and supportive, for instance – but, paradoxically, in doing so, she is endangering the
patients she shows that she sincerely cares for. In impersonating a doctor, her
actions constitute the serious crimes of identity fraud and assault, which carry
lengthy gaol sentences. It is made clear that she is aware of the seriousness of
her actions. In an important scene in Episode 1, "Doctor Ally" must insert an

intercostal catheter to drain blood trapped in a patient's lungs. While Cath knows theoretically what to do, and has witnessed this being performed many times, she had never felt what it was like to carefully punch through fascia and muscles and reach the pleural space. The viewer instinctively knows that both the imposter nurse, acting as doctor, and the real nurse, are present in this moment. While the imposter nurse – now acting as Doctor Ally – must fake her competence, the actual nurse – Nurse Cath – disapproves of the danger in which this puts this patient, making it difficult for Cath/"Ally" to move forward in this procedure.

Another paradox is apparent in how, although there is romance in the narrative, *Trust Me* is not a romantic tale. As a result of her choices, the protagonist loses her innocence regarding the potential for the medical system to be a force for good and participates, albeit initially unwillingly, in the cynicism that surrounds her. In this world, humanity is brutal and justice does not come to the needy. This is an extremely nihilistic view of both health care and the wider world in which it exists. As Hibbs (2011) explains, nihilism suggests that the world *as it ought to be,* does not exist. A nihilistic world is one where rights and dignity, equality and happiness have lost their valued positions, and – in addition – there is a loss of faith in the idea that science and medicine can, and will, resolve problems. In this view, the bases for human existence, including feelings such as suffering, joy and even rage, have no meaning (Nietzsche, 1992).

In Nietzche's influential view, nihilism gives rise to one of two natural reactions: to submit to passivity or be compelled into action. A passive, life-negating reaction is marked by pessimism, emptiness and soulless compliance. According to Nietzsche, individuals in this situation accept subjugation and are on a path to self-destruction. They give up – just as many of the characters in *Trust Me* give in, and give up. In the beginning of the first episode of the series, the hospital's nursing staff express this attitude when they turn a blind eye to obvious medical incompetence, and instead blame an easy victim – the whistleblower, Sister Hardacre.

Conversely, the active reaction establishes a new hierarchy of values – including a will to power. This is itself risky and can lead just as easily to destruction as it can to a more productive life. Cath is consistently shown as taking the active path. She unsuccessfully tries to persuade the management of the hospital in which she works as a nurse to take note of the flaws in their system, then turns to the media to expose the system's shortcomings. In this, she chooses not to accommodate the corrupt status quo, or to stand still and be part of the ongoing decline. But, when she chooses to impersonate a doctor, she also chooses not to adhere to the values that have until that time guided her life – her personal sense of ethics, and the professional medical code of practice and integrity. By impersonating a doctor, she begins down the slippery slope into evil and, along the way, loses her self-respect and, ultimately, her identity. As she states at one point:

When I was a nurse, I saw that things were wrong. That people were dying. I stood up and said so because that's what my dad had always taught me to do and say what was right, not what was easy, and because of that I lost everything. No job. No future for me or my kid. Is that what you get for being a good person? Is that what I deserve? After all the work I've put in.

(third episode)

It is clear, in her constant studying and fear when faced with interventions with which she has no experience, that she is aware of the possible consequences of her lack of knowledge and training, but she continues to maintain her deception, regardless. In contemporary health care, where nurses work in highly technical environments, patients are thought of as cases more than as human beings, and under-resourcing and poor management is a constant theme, nihilism is not unexpected. As McHugh et al. (2011) explain, in such environments, nurses experience excessive work demands and, as a result, frequently expose their patients and themselves to danger. Such nurses can become frustrated that their personal concerns are overlooked in preference for the ever-driving, never-satisfied, needs of increased efficiency and productivity. Many nurses lose heart, become desensitised or operate as if automatically, evolving a form of purely task-oriented working (Fida et al., 2016). In this, they are taking Nietzsche's passive path. Others experience pent up anxiety and anger that converts into diffuse rage that then, often, gets displaced onto other nurses (Evans, Pereira and Parker, 2008). The result is inter-professional conflict, disharmony and petty infighting. Such anger can also affect interactions with patients, or be turned inwards onto the individual nurse themself (Evans, Pereira, and Parker, 2008). Still other nurses give up and leave nursing altogether. Those that remain may, even if they try to stand up to the system, be aware that, in a nihilistic sense, they are fighting a losing and meaningless battle.

Trust Me prompts reflection on what values are needed by nurses as they move from the irreconcilable position of having to tolerate imprudent and destructive policies that depersonalise both patients and healthworkers, to a system that is more enlightened, and functional, yet at that moment unimagined. In a pivotal scene in *Trust Me*, where an elderly woman is being bandaged, "Doctor Ally" excels as a health practitioner because she is able to combine the skills of a nurse such as hugging, bandaging, communicating gently and genuinely caring on a human level, with the role of the doctor, by diagnosing and treating the medical condition of the patient. This, however, while exposing the ideal combination of care and treatment, falls apart because it is not motivated by good intentions. While the patient appreciates the care, and "Doctor Ally's" work is noticed and admired by the nurse on duty, Cath finds the encounter rewarding but also taxing, as she fears exposure.

Although an imposter, with only the outward appearance of professionalism, Cath survives and even thrives as "Ally", despite – and as a result of – her lies.

As such, her character is symbolic of a system that itself only pretends to offer health care and safety. In this system, the truth is disbelieved. When faced with the truth about their hospital, instead of working to remediate the problems, the board attempts to shut down Nurse Cath by suspending her on false charges. Then, when Cath is moved to confess to her neighbour, who is the touchstone of truth and fulfils the role of a surrogate mother in the series, this figure is so trusting that she cannot even comprehend what her friend "Ally" is telling her. As such, *Trust Me* deals powerfully and explicitly with an entrenched problem in health care – the issue of systemic neglect and incompetence. Since incompetence and neglect is being poorly dealt with by the hospital system, *Trust Me* compellingly represents the lengths that some nurses might have to resort to as a consequence. As such, it is a clear and vivid cautionary tale about how lives, and the systems they inhabit and produce, unravel when an ethical pathway is not followed.

Although it is a fictional drama, *Trust Me* (like *Nurse Jackie*) also accurately underscores how tenuously contemporary nurses, as workers, hold on to their standard of living. Many nurses, over ninety percent of whom are women, are also balancing the demands of shift work with parenting and home duties. Yet, nursing work is highly stressful, and not known to be family-friendly (McIntosh et al., 2012). Although now university educated, nurses remain members of the working class, but they no longer have the job security, status or respect the role enjoyed in the past. Their professional situation speaks to that common to many in the twenty-first century who, although employed, live close to the poverty line. As such, nurses are victims of the neoliberalist economic paradigm; where the individual must take responsibility for their own problems, even though society has caused many of them. Heidegger (1954) offers a persuasive critique of blind adherence to the promises of technological progress, arguing that the very essence of technology must be questioned, for it is liable to mire users in a hegemony of instrumentalism (in Krol and Lavoie, 2014, p. 114). Heidegger also warned that technological dependence would take precedence over spirituality, authenticity and creativity in everyday life. In this inauthentic world, characterised by ambiguity and subservience, individuals are rendered empty and passive, again making them vulnerable to nihilism.

Cath is not the only character who succumbs to nihilistic evil and self service in *Trust Me*. The emergency department's male doctor initially appears professional, his self-interest hidden under a veneer of competence and charming attractiveness. When, however, he has to try to resuscitate a six-year-old girl who has been killed after a motor vehicle accident in which she was not wearing a seatbelt, his first response is cynicism. He also displays poor professional/personal boundaries – kissing Cath as the new hire at work and exhibiting other improper behaviour when it suits him. Another character, the senior doctor in the unit, drinks excessively and suffers overwhelming, and paralysing, guilt after the avoidable deaths of patients due to what she feels are her mistakes some years before. Her actions, such as drinking at work, reveals not only that doctors are fallible, but also that she has not learned from the experience. She too is disengaged, cynical and insufficiently focused on her work. The culture of the emergency unit is, itself, similarly corrupt. When a young doctor on the ward tries to create a fair patient allocation system to offset any preferential or improper behaviour, the others jest at his expense. On the other hand, there are vestiges of good practice. There is a nurse character – Nurse Karen, played by Lois Chimimba, who represents the possibility of good practice, but she is also a product of the "sick" system. Hard bitten and wise cracking, she is assertive in a positive way, but also resorts to non-productive eye rolling and openly communicating her feelings of frustration.

Trust Me is compelling viewing due to its clever writing and direction and persuasive acting. It is also arresting because it shines a light on hospital dysfunction. This is in contrast to conventional hospital dramas which emphasise expert problem solving of dramatic health crises and romantic encounters in state-of-the-art facilities. Instead, *Trust Me* can be seen as one of a subgenre of popular contemporary screen narratives exposing institutional mismanagement and abuse. Unfortunately, as a number of contemporary films, such as *Oranges and Sunshine* (Loach, 2010), *Philomena* (Frears, 2013), *The Magdalene Sisters* (Mullan, 2002) and *Spotlight* (McCarthy, 2015), demonstrate, failure within social care systems is not a modern phenomenon. However, not since *The National Health* (Gold, 1973), a British comedy film, has there been a story that has used health service corruption as its subject matter in such a forthright and sustained manner. In reality, though, scandalous complaints of incompetence, abuse, neglect and non-accountability have triggered reviews of hospitals and other institutional care systems across the Western world for many decades (Rafter et al., 2014).

No place of asylum

There is no better embodiment of the demise of the once-idealised "modern" health care institution – where patients could receive lengthy hospitalisation ranging from acute treatment to rehabilitation, constant care from qualified nurses and doctors, and a gentle re-introduction into the community – than the mental asylum (Bachrach, 1984). Mental asylums were originally established to offer sanctuary to the most vulnerable members of the community, those who had been outcast and neglected because of fear, ignorance and beliefs that mental illness was incurable or contagious (Carrier and Tomlinson, 2003). During, and following, the Industrial Revolution, the specialist training of psychiatric doctors and nurses and the development of dedicated mental institutions expanded greatly. Large institutions with the capacity to hold thousands of patients were built, and operated initially on a custodial model, in which patients were largely meant to live out their lives in a home-like and secure environment, which was, however, separated from society (Chow and Priebe, 2013). As well as strict supervision and set routines, innovative treatments such as hydrotherapy, electric therapies, sedating medications and occupational strategies were used to manage and treat patients. However, the Great Depression and the two world wars soon saw the depletion of staff and resources from these asylums, and patients' needs became secondary to those of the general population and the war-effort (Barton, 1998). Management of patients became stricter, as fewer staff struggled to cope with meagre resources and over-crowding.

The direness of this care is vividly portrayed in Mary Jane Ward's semi-autobiographical novel, *The Snake Pit*, published in 1946, and Litvak's 1948 film adapted from it. Although over seventy years old, this book and film remain horrifying, realistic and significant exposés of the deplorable conditions that people with mental distress suffered in this period. Well received by critics (Howard Gotleib Archival Research Centre n.d.), *The Snake Pit* was a Book of the Month Club choice, excerpted in *Harper's Bazaar*, condensed in *The Readers Digest* and translated into five languages. It was so popular with readers that it established what was then called a "madness fashion" in literature (E.P. 1946, p. 15), with publishers releasing many other novels about mental illness to meet this demand. Closely based on the book, but with some changes to translate the story to the screen, the film opened in New York in 1948 and then in other parts of the world the following year. The film was also extrememly successful, grossing $US4.1 million in ticket sales, placing it equal second in 1949 US/Canadian box-office sales (Reid, 2010, p. 301) and being nominated for six Academy Awards.

The film begins with a deceptively tranquil garden scene. A young woman, Virginia (played by Olivia de Havilland), is seated alone on a bench. Disembodied voices are heard, and she tries to make sense of the strange experience. This sets an important tone for viewers – they are about to enter the subjective, and closed, world of mental illness, a liminal space where horrific experiences befall Virginia and the other patients. Instead of normal life, this is a "madhouse" – a home where the unhomely reigns and where uncanny experiences are common. Litvak made use of a then-innovative camera panning technique in this film called the "whip pan", which zoomed in, out and around to scan a wide scene. This procedure brought to filmic life the magnitude of disturbed behaviour, crowded conditions and inescapable torment. There are also scenes that present much of life in such asylums as taxing and terrifying. From treatments that involved hours of immersion in hot or cold water baths, "unmodified" ElectroConvulsiveTherapy (ECT) (administered without anaesthetic or muscle relaxant) and sedation-induced sleep during which patients were rendered helpless, to hunger and boredom, everything was made more frightening due to living in close quarters with large numbers of severely disturbed patients. This fear is further suggested through the use of filmic conventions redolent of earlier expressionist horror films like *Nosferatu* (Murnau, 1922) and *The Cabinet of Dr. Caligari* (Weine, 1920), such as the use of black and white film stock, extensive use of extreme close-up camera angles, lighting that cast long shadows, and heavy-handed dramatic metaphors, including the emblematic snake pit scene when a throng of patients metamorphoses into a mass of writhing snakes trapped at the bottom of a dark pit. The black and white film stock emphasises the binary contrast between sanity and insanity, and the inner workings of the mind and outer reality, and plays up the vulnerable innocence of de Havilland's pale shining beauty.

In 2002, Clooney nominated the film as one of the "movies that changed us" in his influential book of that title. In the late 1940s, the response to the film was so robust and compelling that, as a result of discussions around the issue, twenty-six American states eventually changed their mental health laws and instituted the policy of deinstitutionalisation, which was later also later introduced in the UK, Australia and New Zealand. Large institutions were gradually replaced with community-based care and small hospital units that focused more on democratic principles and openness. This situation was also critically exposed in photo-documentaries such as those by Albert Maisel (1946) and scholarly commentaries such as Erving Goffman's *Asylum* (1961), however, it was the film of *The Snake Pit* which brought this issue to light and focused public notice on a mass scale. While today the book is relatively unexplored as a literary work, the enduring power of the film of *The Snake Pit* in relation to the representation of mental illness and its treatment is evidenced by the number of articles in medical journals that use it in an analysis of the history, and accuracy, of the portrayal of mental illness on screen (see, for example, Atkinson, 2005; Dowbiggin, 2013; Grob, 1994). The film has also been included in numerous popular culture-focused studies of gender, sexism and mental illness in film (see, Fishbein, 1979; Semarne, 1994).

The Snake Pit articulates widely held fears about insanity at a time when mental illness was thought to be incurable, and some years before antipsychotic medications became widely accessible (López-Muñoz et al., 2005). The formidable nurse characters are a key aspect in conjuring the horror – they are stern, detached, and lacking any empathy or kindness. The floridly psychotic and seriously disturbed Virginia nevertheless recovers despite the quite grotesque obstacles placed in her path. These obstacles are institutional and include the asylum's overcrowded and mind-numbing physical environs, a lack of empathy from staff, poor hygiene, under-nutrition and often being cold, bored and, at times, caged like an animal. Although by the end of the book Virginia feels strong enough to leave the asylum, she is also aware that many remain trapped behind her. These are not only hapless and vulnerable patients, but also the traumatised nurses and doctors who tend to them. To make this point, the book ends with a chilling image: as Virginia is readying to leave the asylum, she performs a number of rituals that reflect her liberation from institutionalisation. She tears her name and number out of her coat, and reclaims the fine linen handkerchiefs that have been kept from her. Two nurses, Sommerville and Vance, complete their final assessment of the soon-to-be-discharged patient. At this time, it becomes clear that Nurse Sommerville has, herself, become seriously disturbed as a result of working in the asylum. The deplorable conditions, constant noise, threats, and sheer weight of patient numbers and work to be done have traumatised her, taking her beyond her coping abilities and she has decompensated. Driven into insanity, Nurse Sommerville has fallen from the position of nurse in charge to an incurable mental patient. The image of the nurse-as-patient upsets the normal order of the world and reinforces the damage inherent in the asylum's daily routine. While the issue of second victim syndrome has been discussed in nursing literature (Seys et al., 2013), rarely has this been portrayed on film. Second victim phenomenon is the appearance of emotional shock after a person has witnessed a traumatic clinical incident. Such incidents, even though they may not directly involve a "victim" can be traumatising because the danger and unexpectedness is so shocking. Unfortunately, unprovoked violence, extreme distress or multiple patient traumas are common in some nursing contexts such as emergency departments and mental health settings (Scott et al., 2010).

If no one looks, does anyone see?

Calls for more enlightenened and humane treatment of mental illness have not abated since systems of mental health care were established (Stanley and Manthorpe, 2001). In the late twentieth century in Australia, mental health care that was supposed to be a model of innovation suffered similar critique in the mainstream media, exposed through a *60 Minutes* special episode (Harvey and Taylor, 1988), after years of persistent lobbying from a patient advocacy group. "Ward 10B" situated in Townsville Hospital in northern Queensland, Australia, was the first unit in that state to operationalise the concept of a "therapeutic community". This model of care first developed in Britain after the second world war. There, it was found that groups of returned prisoners of war were better able to adapt back into civilian society in an environment that was more democratic – paying more attention to patients' opinions – and where authoritarian and controlling practices were avoided (Harrison, 2000). The central philosophy of a therapeutic community is that patients (known as "clients") are active participants in their own, and each other's, mental health treatment and that responsibility for the daily running of the community is shared among the clients and the staff (Manning, 2013). In this model, the power differential between clients and the nurses and doctors is reduced and the clients discuss and vote on daily approaches to care for individuals and the group. Successful therapeutic communities tend to be those where the client-base shares many similarities (for example, all clients are drug dependant), because a wide understanding of symptoms is achievable (Manning, 2013).

Drawing on this innovative model, the nursing staff in Ward 10B worked in ways that contrasted markedly with their more traditional peers who worked in hospitals such as Wolston Park in Brisbane or in large asylums like those represented in *The Snake Pit*. Nurses working at Wolston Park generally conformed to the medical model of care – wearing traditional white uniforms, the nurses worked in teams to ensure basic needs such as food, hygiene and safety needs were met. They provided firm limits on abnormal behaviours and assisted with treatments such as administering medications and the delivery of ECT, occupational therapy and health education. Nurses in Ward 10B, however, wore plain clothes (presumably to blend with the clients and moderate class differentials) and took a "hands-off" approach to such aspects of care as bed-making and hygiene routines (Alchin and Weatherhead, 1976). Instead, they facilitated discussion groups with clients, were laissez-faire about idiosyncratic behaviours, and only dispensed medications and other treatments when the group decided these actions were to be taken. In some cases, this liberal approach was effective, particularly if the clients were lucid and motivated. Townsville Hospital was, however, a large general public hospital that accepted patients exhibiting a wide range of mental disorders from anxiety and postnatal depression through to florid psychosis and suicidality. Many had co-morbid conditions that required individualised and expert assessment and care, and could not be appropriately managed using a group consensus approach. Ward 10B was also, like most Australian mental health services at the time, chronically understaffed in terms of the numbers of nurses and their areas of expertise (Alavi and Frow, 1991).

Complaints about Ward 10B began in 1975, just two years after the experiment had begun (Carter, 1991). It was to take another decade, and more than a hundred complaints, however, for anything to be done. Far from a progressive and innovative model of care, Ward 10B was characterised by the use of heavy-handed and rigid interaction, poor clinical judgment and outdated treatments. Staff, however, considered their techniques revolutionary (Ellard, 1991; Wilson, 2003). A carer action group, frustrated with the lack of responsiveness from the Health Department, repeatedly lobbied the media. Eventually, they were successful in attracting national exposure when the high profile Australian television current affairs programme *60 Minutes* (Harvey and Taylor, 1988) ran a story about the abuse. Finally, the Health Minister was pressured into taking action and the State Government established a Commission of Inquiry. The commissioner, William Carter Q.C., heard testimony from many patients, carers and staff including nurses, and found that patients in the ward were subjected to verbal and physical abuse, experienced severe restrictions on their civil liberty, and that the principles of a therapeutic community were rigidly applied without regard for individual circumstances. Sensational newspaper headlines captured the attention of the Queensland public, and have entered the mythology of fear around instutionalisation for mental illness. The case of the anonymised "Patient 31" detailed in the Commission of Inquiry's report is a typical example of what went wrong:

P31 was a psychotic patient who was also dying of acute brain syndrome. On 23 February 1987, one of the doctors at the unit noted in her file that she reported feeling alone and was terrified of dying. In spite of this she was still required to attend daily group meetings. One day, because she had been screaming all morning, the staff psychologist moved that the patient would only be allowed to speak in the group if she spoke "in a high [pitched] voice" which she refused to do. This was typical of group therapy at the ward. (Queensland Commission of Inquiry, Report, 9.3.138)

In 1991, the Commissioner identified sixty-five deaths relevant to the inquiry, including twenty-seven suicides linked to ward practices (Wilson, 2003). In these cases, patients had informed nursing and other staff of their intentions, had indicated suicidality prior to admission, lacked proper diagnosis and treatment, or were discharged without any risks being communicated to others. Other scandalous treatment was revealed: patients received heavy doses of barbiturates (a drug then no longer used in mental health) to keep them sedated; a baby was kept in a suitcase rather than a cot; patients were left lying in urine-soaked beds for days; and, patients made clinical decisions that related to other patients. Finally, Carter determined that the care and treatment of patients at Townsville Hospital was negligent, unsafe, unethical and unlawful. The unit was eventually closed, a few state-based Health Department officials were demoted, and the therapeutic community model was proscribed through Queensland, but not before the unit's charismatic and popular director, Dr. John Lindsay, had retired to write a book on the affair. In this, he termed the scrutiny a "witch-hunt" (Lindsay, 1992) and urged loyal nursing staff to resist changing their practice.

Paradoxically, Ward 10B's vision of being progressive, democratic and user-led turned out to be repressive and rigid in practice. The nurses who worked there adopted an almost cult-like adherence to eccentric processes, which were out of touch with contemporary standards and practices, and denied rights to patients and their families. In an attempt to break free of a dominating medical discourse that was characteristic of the old asylums, the staff of Ward 10B only succeeded in creating a domination of a different form. A therapeutic community begins with the premise of complete openness, yet this was a closed system with impervious boundaries. Despite the amount of popular press and mass media devoted to the scandal, there is, depressingly, no evidence that systemic changes have been put into place to prevent such a situation occuring again. As De Maria and Jan (1996) state:

The inquiry also found evidence of widespread patient abuse, head-office cover-ups, and criminal negligence. In fact, it is fair to say that the inquiry exposed the worst identified psychiatric atrocity in Queensland's mental health history. Again, we must say that no charges have been laid and no process of ethical renewal has been undertaken within the psychiatric system. The system remains ready to generate new forms of psychiatric wrongdoing.

(p. 155)

At least some nurses working in this unit, or winessing these abuses, also clearly had misgivings about the practices and their effects. Yet no one felt able to step forward and articulate these reservations. This is a clear case of a system in which nurses contributed to its dysfunction and were not agents of positive change. They had the power to stop the illegal activities and to provide compassionate care and yet they did not. They also remained unrepentant and felt misunderstood. In this way, their collective dark side – a propensity for corruption and evil – was denied or suppressed. In a Jungian view, these were individuals who had not been able to integrate their propensity for both good and bad beliefs and behaviour.

Conclusion

Almost forty years ago, Beardshaw (1981) wrote about nurses standing up for what they believe is right:

> What I saw was wrong and should have been reported. You've got to look ahead – one day you might be a patient. You set the standards – you've got to set the standards. It was on my conscience all the time – it's got to be reported. In the end I did it, and only when I did it did I feel happy. Otherwise you feel a part of it, as much to blame. I would have felt I had committed a greater crime had I not reported it.
>
> (p. 28)

It is, however, a depressing reality that cases of neglect and poor standards of care continue to occur within health services (Andrews and Butler, 2014; Francis, 2013; Gosport; 2018; World Health Organization, 2005). The risk for whistle-blowing in any organisation, but particularly in nursing, is that there will be reprisals for the whistleblower, and this is the background to *Trust Me*. Another reality about whistleblowing is that it can expose dysfunction, but not repair it. This issue is reflected in the story of Ward 10B. Since nurses make up the vast majority of staff working in the health professions (WHO, 2017), it is essential that they are aware, firstly, that bad practice occurs and, secondly, of how to speak up in a way that is both clear and safe, so that improvements can be made, patients can be well cared for, and the whistleblower themselves does not suffer reprisals.

Apart from providing general health care, nurses can play a role in improving health inequities by engaging with, and influencing, marginalised individuals and communities. Their trustworthiness, patient accessibility and health knowledge are valued resources that allow them to help vulnerable people, such as those living with mental illness or from minority cultures, and who experience disadvantage because of stigma and a lack of understanding (Lauder et al., 2006). Nurses can, therefore, be key agents for social change. But professional advancement and participation as social activists requires long term commitment. Nursing's advancement and strong professional identity requires a long game – a long game wherein the public is presented with nursing's complexities and diversity, and where nurses acknowledge that their role is social and political and they need to be accountable for their actions and empowered professionals.

References

Alavi C and Frow J (1991) Firm judgments on uncertain issues *Australian Society* August 19–20.

Alchin S and Weatherhead R (1976) *Psychiatric Nursing: A Practical Approach.* Sydney: McGraw-Hill.

Andrews J and Butler M (2014) *Trusted to care: An independent review of the Princess of Wales Hospital and Neath Port Talbot Hospital at Abertawe Bro Morgannwg University Health Board.* Available at: https://gov.wales/sites/default/files/publications/2019-04/trusted-to-care.pdf.

Atkinson R (2005) Revisiting a classic: *The Snake Pit Clinical Psychiatry News* 33(8): 21–22.

Bachrach L (1984) Asylum and chronically ill psychiatric patients *American Journal of Psychiatry* 141(8): 975–978.

Barton W (1998) A history of psychiatry: From the era of the asylum to the age of Prozac *Psychiatric Services* 49(9): 1241–1242.

Beardshaw V (1981). *Conscientious Objectors at Work: Mental Hospital Nurses: A Case Study.* London: Social Audit.

Calkin S (2011) Whistleblowing Mid Staffs nurse too scared to walk to car after shift. *Nursing Times* 7 October. Available at: www.nursingtimes.net/clinical-archive.

Carrier J and Tomlinson D (2003) *Asylum in the Community.* New York: Routledge.

Carter H (1991) *Report of the Commission of Inquiry into the Care and Treatment of Consumers in the Psychiatric Unit (Ward 10B) of the Townsville General Hospital.* Brisbane: Australian Government Printing Service.

Chow W and Priebe S (2013) Understanding psychiatric institutionalization: A conceptual review *BMC Psychiatry* 13(1): art 169.

Clooney N (2002) *The Movies that Changed Us: Reflections on a Screen.* New York: Atria.

De Maria W and Jan C (1996) Behold the shut eyed sentry! Whistleblower perspectives on government failure to correct wrongdoing *Crime, Law & Social Change* 24: 151–166.

Dowbiggin I (2013) *The Quest for Mental Health: A Tale of Science, Medicine, Scandal, Sorrow, and Mass Society.* Cambridge: Cambridge University Press.

E P (1946) Literary development of Rumer Godden *The Argus* 21: September 15.

Ellard J (1991) The lessons from Townsville *Modern Medicine* 34(7): 34–38.

Evan M (1999) *The Impostor Phenomenon: A Descriptive Study of Its Incidence among Registered Nurse Preceptors.* Lubbock: Texas Technical University.

Evans A, Pereira D and Parker J (2008) Discourses of anxiety in nursing practice: A psychoanalytic case study of the change-of-shift handover ritual *Nursing Inquiry* 15(1): 40–48.

Fida R, Tramontano C, Paciello M, Kangasniemi M, Sili A, Bobbio A and Barbaranelli C (2016) Nurse moral disengagement *Nursing Ethics* 23(5): 547–564.

Fishbein L (1979) *The Snake Pit* (1948): The sexist nature of sanity *American Quarterly* 31(5): 641–665.

Francis R (2013) *Report of the Mid Staffordshire NHS Foundation Trust Public Inquiry: Executive Summary*. London: The Stationery Office.

Frears S (dir) (2013) *Philomena*. Film. Hollywood: Weinstein.

Goffman E (1961) *Asylum*. New York: Anchor Books.

Gold J (dir) (1973) *The National Health*. Film. London: Virgin Films.

Gosport Independent Panel (2018) *Gosport War Memorial Hospital: The Report of the Gosport Independent Panel*. London: Department of Health. Available at: www.gosportpanel.inde pendent.gov.uk/media/documents/070618_CCS207_CCS03183220761_Gosport_In quiry_Whole_Document.pdf.

Gough P (1998) UKCC review: Talking back. Nurses have risen to the challenges posed in the draft review of nursing regulation says Pippa Gough. Sue Norman expands on bogus nurses, one of the many issues raised by the UKCC in its response. And GP Ian Banks warns against the review's suggestion of a single regulatory body for all health professionals *Nursing Standard* 12(28): 16–17.

Grob G (1994) *Mad Among Us*. New York: Simon and Schuster.

Harrison T (2000) *Bion, Rickman, Foulkes, and the Northfield Experiments: Advancing on a Different Front, Vol 5*. London: Jessica Kingsley Publishers.

Harvey G and Taylor S (1988) *Ward 10B*. VHS. Sydney: Nine Network.

Heidegger M (1954) *Essais et Conférences*. Paris: Gallimard, Mesnil Sur l'Éstrée.

Hibbs T (2011) *Shows about Nothing: Nihilism in Popular Culture*. Waco: Baylor University Press.

Howard Gotleib Archival Research Centre (n.d.) Ward, Mary Jane (1905–1981). Boston University: Howard Gotleib Archival Research Centre. Available at: http://hgar-srv3.bu.edu/collections/collection?id=122935.

Krol P and Lavoie M (2014) Beyond nursing nihilism, a Nietzschean transvaluation of neoliberal values *Nursing Philosophy* 15: 112–124.

Lauder W, Reel S, Farmer J and Griggs H (2006) Social capital, rural nursing and rural nursing theory *Nursing Inquiry* 13(1): 73–79.

Lindsay J (1992) *The Deadly Witch-hunt*. Main Beach: Wileman Publications.

Loach J (dir) (2010) *Oranges and Sunshine*. Film. London: BBC.

López-Muñoz F, Alamo C, Cuenca E, Shen W, Clervoy P and Rubio G (2005) History of the discovery and clinical introduction of chlorpromazine *Annals of Clinical Psychiatry* 17(3): 113–135.

Maisel A (1946) Bedlam 1946: Most of U.S mental hospitals are a shame and disgrace *Life Magazine* 6: May 102–118.

Manning N (2013) *The Therapeutic Community Movement: Charisma and Routinisation*. London: Routledge.

McAllister M and Brien D L (2015) Looking back to see ahead: Reassessing *The Snake Pit* for its Gothic codes and significance. In *Peer Reviewed Proceedings: 6th Annual Conference, Popular Culture Association of Australia and New Zealand (popcaanz)*. Wellington: Popular Culture Association of Australia and New Zealand, 84–94.

McCarthy T (dir) (2015) *Spotlight*. Film. Hollywood: Participant Media.

McHugh M, Kutney-Lee A, Cimiotti J, Sloane D and Aiken L (2011) Nurses' widespread job dissatisfaction, burnout, and frustration with health benefits signal problems for patient care *Health Affairs* 30(2): 202–210.

McIntosh B, McQuaid R, Munro A and Dabir-Alai P (2012) Motherhood and its impact on career progression *Gender in Management: An International Journal* 27(5): 346–364.

Mullan P (dir) (2002) *The Magdalene Sisters*. Film. Edinburgh: Miramax.

Murnau F (dir) (1922) *Nosferatu*. Film. Weimar Republic: Film Arts Guild.

Murray T, Philipsen N, Brice E, Harvin L, Hinds D and Warren-Dorsey R (2011) Health care fraud: Stopping nurse imposters *The Journal for Nurse Practitioners* 7(9): 753–760.

Nietzsche F (1992) Beyond good and evil. In Kaufmann W (ed) *The Basic Writings of Nietzsche*. New York: Random House, 179–435.

Poulsen J (2016) Darwin man Nicholas Crawford convicted and fined for claiming to be a nurse. *NT News* 5 October. Available at: www.ntnews.com.au/news/northern-territory/darwin-man-nicholas-crawford-convicted-and-fined-for-claiming-to-be-a-nurse/news-story/968cc38beb0e8e20b27bcd7e9071f177.

Rafter N, Hickey A, Condell S, Conroy R, O'Connor P, Vaughan D and Williams D (2014) Adverse events in healthcare: Learning from mistakes *QJM: An International Journal of Medicine* 108(4): 273–277.

Reid J (2010) *Hollywood Classics: Title Index to All Movies Reviewed in Books*. Morrisville: Lulu Press.

Scott S, Hirschinger L, Cox K, McCoig M, Hahn-Cover K, Epperly K, Phillips E and Hall L (2010) Caring for our own: Deploying a systemwide second victim rapid response team *The Joint Commission Journal on Quality and Patient Safety* 36(5): 233–240.

Semarne V (1994) *The Snake Pit*: A woman's serpentine journey toward (w)holeness *Literature/Film Quarterly* 22(3): 144–150.

Seys D, Wu A, Gerven E, Vleugels A, Euwema M, Panella M and Vanhaecht K (2013) Health care professionals as second victims after adverse events: A systematic review *Evaluation & The Health Professions* 36(2): 135–162.

Stanley N and Manthorpe J (2001) Reading mental health inquiries: Messages for social work *Journal of Social Work* 1(1): 77–99.

Wallaston S (2017) *Trust Me* review – Jodie Whittaker is warm and watchable as a fake doctor (not that Doctor). *The Guardian* 9 August. Available at: www.theguardian.com/tv-and-radio/2017/aug/09/trust-me-review-jodie-whittaker-doctor.

Weine R (dir) (1920) *The Cabinet of Doctor Caligari*. Film. Weimar Republic: Decla-Bioscop.

Wilson E (2003) 'Eccentric and idiosyncratic treatment philosophies': The therapeutic community at Townsville's Ward 10B, Queensland, 1973–87 *Health and History* 5(2): 60–74.

World Health Organization (2017) *The 2017 Update*. Global Health Workforce Statistics Geneva: World Health Organization.

9 Growing from adversity

Introduction

One way of viewing nursing is to see the profession as a cultural group that has developed over time and, throughout this history, been controlled and regulated. Always-pressing concerns keep nurses focused on the present, too busy to look back, too pressured to look forward. As a consequence, many nurses today lack an awareness of their professional origins and cannot confidently articulate either individual or collective nursing values. This chapter explores aspects of nursing's repression, as well as its resilience, using some key stories in popular culture which illuminate aspects of nursing that are not often discussed in professional forums.

The gendered and religious history of nursing – in which ideas of duty and servitude are strongly present – have shaped how the nursing profession is perceived by the public including those in the media and artists, as well as by health care colleagues and nurses themselves (Traynor and Evans, 2014). This is dramatically illustrated in a scene from the classic film *The Nun's Story* (Zinnemann, 1959). In this strikingly beautiful film shot in black and white, based on the bestselling novel of the same name by Kathryn Hulme (1956), Audrey Hepburn plays a nun, Sister Luke, who is also a nurse. Struggling with her vocation, Sister Luke is judged by her superior as lacking in humility. In order that she can learn a lesson in self-effacement, she is sent to work in an insane asylum. There, she is witness to brutal treatments and introduced to what the nursing supervisor describes as "the violent cases". As they approach a treatment room, this nurse provides Sister Luke with a summary of what she will find inside,

> We keep them in baths maintained at a constant temperature. The sound that you hear are their heels beating up and down against the tubs. Sister Marie is on duty. She generally remains there from eight to ten hours at a time.

Although Sister Luke nods, she is speechless. A heavy door is opened to release a cacophony of screaming, pleading and weeping. The steam dissipates to reveal several patients lying in full-length baths, restrained by canvas covers. A solitary nurse is seated in the far corner. So that she can be heard above the terrible wailing, the Senior Sister loudly announces Sister Luke's name. But the solitary nurse, Sister Marie, has no time to acknowledge her, as she is called to one of the patients, who is begging for water to quench her thirst. Wide-eyed, Sister Luke takes in the horrifying scene as she is given a handwritten order from the senior nurse that reads: "You will be Sister Marie's assistant here". In response, Sister Luke nods humbly.

In this scene, the patient is a symbol of otherness (Foucault, 2005), referred to only as "them" and its derivatives. The nurse, in accepting an allocation for which she is unprepared, and bearing witness to cruel treatments because she feels duty-bound by her vocational calling, plays out her own subordinate position in a rigid hierarchy. This is an identity that is strengthened by a belief in doing good for the world through obedience (Nelson, 2010). But, as the narrative progresses, Sister Luke is seen to struggle with an inner conflict between the rules of her congregation and her desire to bring about systemic change; this conflict manifesting, therefore, between her role as a group member and that of an autonomous person. Despite the insistent subjugation and the terrible conditions of the institution, Sister Luke is not broken by the demands that are placed upon her. Instead, she provides the best care possible to her patients by being empathic and compassionate, praying for strength, sublimating her anxieties into hard work, and acknowledging to her supervisor that she needs support. These are examples of pragmatic solutions to her inner struggle. The nun's story is about personal transformation, and a metaphor for how nurses can grow from adversity.

Transcending personal trauma

Aside from dealing with the traumas of others, nurses can also bring their own personal traumas to their work. In the novel *The English Patient* (Ondaatje, 1993) and film made from it (Minghella, 1996), protagonist Nurse Hana has been traumatised by the gruelling experiences of war and has, in a sense, become imprisoned by torturous emotions that are too confronting for her to manage. Aside from encountering patients who are suffering excruciating agony from devastating and often incurable wounds, she endures the death of her father and fiancé. Then, when the truck in which she is travelling triggers a landmine, she narrowly survives an explosion that kills several colleagues. As a result of these crushing difficulties, she is barely able to function as either a nurse or as a person, and instead cannot do other than perfunctorily complete her nursing tasks and interactions. While superficially appearing efficient and dedicated, something important is missing from her life and work. She has faced a demon – the machinery of war – and this has destroyed her psychologically, to the extent where she feels incapable of re-entering her own life. When a badly burnt patient who would be unlikely to survive a planned road trip is identified, she volunteers to stay behind the unit in a ruined villa, to care for him. On one level, this is a way for her to avoid the inevitable –

confronting her losses and returning home to Canada in her damaged state. However, on another level, the enforced isolation in the villa provides an opportunity for her transformation.

As the days pass, Hana engages in a series of mundane experiences, a number in the company of Almasy, the burned man, the so-called "English Patient". In her care of him, as well as in her various exploratory ramblings through the ruins of the gardens, library and chapel, and her encounters with the mine sweeper Kip and the thief Caravaggio, she begins to be able to access her own feelings. Experiencing the true meanings of altruism, kindness, compassion, humility and love, she then feeds these emotions into her actions as a nurse. Instead of treating Almasy in the coolly efficient way she has nursed others, she sits with him and listens deeply as he reminisces about his life. She comforts him in his pain, bathes his wounds and reads to him from a book that interests him. This connection allows Almasy to make peace with what has happened to him and prepare for death. Ceasing to treat her patient in a detached manner, she begins to care for him by learning about his uniqueness, recognising his personal strengths and responding to his needs. As Hana also becomes strong enough to begin to grieve her own losses, she learns to once again find meaning and joy in life and readies herself to re-enter her world outside the villa. Hana is a wounded healer.

Wounded healers

The wounded healer is an archetypal figure who is often discussed within nursing and health. Wounded healers are caregivers who are themselves damaged but, paradoxically, learn to use their suffering to help others (Conti-O'Hare, 2002; Heinrich, 1992). The wounded healer is based on the Greek mythological figure of Chiron, renowned for his medical powers, but also suffering an incurable wound inflicted from an arrow shot by Hercules (Dunn, 2000). Applied by Jung and later therapists as a component of psychoanalysis, the idea of the wounded healer is underpinned by the recognition that a healer can be more effective if they develop an awareness of their past wounds and use this vulnerability to connect, and empathise, with their patients.

The wounded healer appears several times within *The English Patient*. The figure can be recognised in Almasy himself, a man who has suffered both betrayal and physical trauma, but who has something important to teach his vulnerable nurse. It has been suggested that Almasy is like the mythological Fisher King (Fledderus, 1997). In Arthurian legend, the Fisher King is the last keeper of the Holy Grail – an object that offers happiness and wellbeing (Loomis, 1991). But the Fisher King is also suffering from a mysterious and disabling injury, suggesting that although he can reach out to help others, he cannot cure himself. Caravaggio is also a wounded healer. During the war he uses his skills as a thief to spy for the military, but has both thumbs cut off during Nazi interrogation. In talking to Hana, he enables her to tell her story and thus becomes a catalyst for her change. Nunan (2011) suggests that the landscape itself acts as a wounded healer – the ravaged and looted villa is littered with mines, the fields are barren and untended and yet, even in this damaged place, there is shelter, trees producing fruit and frescoes to admire. In particular, the library offers a portal for recovery, with its books providing a comforting escape for the villa's inhabitants. Itself wounded, the library adjusts to bomb damage and is thus still able to offer comfort to its visitors: "The rest of the room had adapted itself to this wound [a hole in the roof], accepting the habits of weather, evening stars, the sound of birds" (Ondaatje, 1993, p. 12).

Hana only becomes aware of how damaged she is when she meets Almasy. With his burns, bandages and abject grief, he is the epitome of the faceless, unknowable and lost patients she had repeatedly and anonymously referred to as "Buddy". In him, she sees herself, he functions as "a pool for her" (Ondaatje, 1993, p. 44). Rather than just dispensing formalised superficial care as she had become very expert in doing, in caring for this sole patient, she begins to feel safer and to grow into herself as a human, as well as a nurse:

> she felt safe here, half adult and half child. Coming out of what had happened to her during the war, she drew her own few rules to herself. She would not be ordered again or carry out duties for the greater good. She would care only for the burned patient. She would read to him and bathe him and give him his doses of morphine.
>
> (Ondaatje, 1993, p. 15)

As the story progresses, the nurse Hana experiences growth from trauma, and is able to use her own woundedness to connect and empathise with her patient. In the process of caring for him in a more present, personalised and compassionate way, she also finds a path to her own personal health and happiness. In this regard, Hana has reached a state of self-actualisation, and her future holds a promise of fulfilment and happiness (McAllister, 2017).

As a holistic practice, nursing relies not only on competence in terms of clinical skills, but also on the ability of nurses to empathise and show compassion. However, it also must be recognised that nursing is a highly stressful and draining profession. As for Hana, it can seem easier for nurses to engage with patients in a routinised, objective manner, maintaining a barrier between themselves and the people for whom they are caring. In many instances, such detachment is fostered by both external, as well as internal, forces. Strong cultural practices can develop amongst nurses where neophytes are admonished to keep a distance from patients if they are seen to come too close, an attitude which is furthered by the highly bureaucratic system in which nurses work. An individual nurse can enter the profession full of desire to empathise with, and care for, patients in a compassionate way but then find themselves overwhelmed by the raw and bloody nature their work, and the mandates of the organisation in which they are operating. In these circumstances, it is easy to give up ideals and seek the security of routine (Sharp, McAllister and Broadbent, 2015). The idea that nurses can be more effective if they can overcome these obstacles, by connecting with the concept of the wounded healer has been explored by researchers (Corso, 2012; Hall, 1997; Paul, 1985) who have also commented on the barriers that exist between nurses and their ability to provide compassionate, empathic care for patients. Corso comments, for example, that the "healing that flows from a clinician who is mindful of her or his own fragility and brokenness is, for many patients, the balm needed to ease suffering, diminish anxiety, and offer solace" (2012, p. 449).

In caring for the patient, Hana ultimately finds her own redemption. As Haswell and Edwards state (2004, p. 130), "in this refuge she is able to find the means to care again about others ... it is the patient who draws her back into a human community". The relevance of this transformation for nurses more generally is that adversity should be expected, and nurses need to be self-aware enough to prepare for it and then gain from engaging with such difficulty. Hana shows nurses that, in facing challenges, change is possible and beneficial. Her story also reveals how self-awareness can help a nurse to return to their authentic self and reclaim authentic values.

From slave to "stronger than the enemy"

Another story set in the past, the film *Paradise Road* (Beresford, 1997), dramatises the true-life experiences of a group of captured nurses (and other women) following the fall of Singapore. The director, Bruce Beresford, based the film on the diaries that Sister Betty Jeffrey kept during the time of her imprisonment, published as *White Coolies* (1954), and the oral testimonies of fellow internee Sister Vivian Bullwinkel and other Japanese Prisoner of War survivors. The women in this jungle internment camp represent many races and positions in society, and include Australian army nurses, Dutch women who had been living in the East Indies, English women from Singapore, Catholic nuns, missionaries and others from diverse nations. Despite this multiplicity, they are all enslaved and have their bodies and spirits profoundly tested. Yet, they also find creative ways to resist their oppressors and the oppression under which they are suffering. In learning to survive, they teach themselves how to transcend the enemy, in the process revealing that their nemesis is not just the Japanese army. It is also their own initial sense of themselves as victims, as well as their defeatist beliefs and inability to work together. In response, they begin to enact resistance practices, which also emphasise their own humanity. Captured and imprisoned, they endure deprivation and harsh treatment before being freed three years later when the Japanese surrender. Apart from the fascinating history it relates, *Paradise Road* is one of the few popular narratives where nurses are represented as a group rather than (a series of) individuals. This is, moreover, a group that is tested in a crisis and that responds collectively in innovative and inspiring ways. In contrast also to other stories of resilience, the nurses in this film do not turn inward and focus on themselves (McAllister, 2014). Instead, they turn to each other for support and, in doing so, find that their united strength is what helps each person deal with the adversity they face. As such, this becomes a narrative about how small, repeated, externally focused oppositional practices enable individuals to cope with trauma, and assist them to reclaim some sense of power and stop seeing themselves as victims.

Although the women are culturally divided – there are language, religious, political and social barriers – they make a decision early in their imprisonment to look out for one another. In one powerful scene, after defying an order to be silent, Nurse Susan Macarthy (played by Cate Blanchett) is forced to kneel under the blaze of the tropical sun for many hours. She is humiliated, demoralised and, in her already weakened state, pushed to her limits. But, upon her release, she is immediately tended to by her comrades. She is fed, cleaned and her wounds are dressed. Others take on her duties until she is well again. In another scene, when the group is starving and forced to eat rancid rice, one of the women catches a snake in the paddy field and the others help to cook it and distribute the result. When one is rewarded with a gift of soap, she shares it with the others and, in this way, when one woman benefits, they all do. Individually, they are all weak and vulnerable, but each gains strength by sharing their work and any bounty. The film is also unusual in not depicting a single dominant leader of the group, with numerous characters demonstrating leadership skills that meet the others' physical and emotional needs. For example, one Dutch woman, who is clearly well educated and of a higher class than many of the others, uses her cunning to barter with the guards and secure medicines, food and alcohol for general use. The trust and honest communication are, however, hard won, as illustrated in a scene of conflict, when the group threatens to divide. This occurs when the younger and more attractive women are invited to live in the Japanese officer's club where they will enjoy good food and clean rooms with hot water, in return for providing the men with sexual favours. Many of the women are horrified and repulsed by this offer, but some find it too tempting to refuse. Instead of causing irreparable fragmentation in the group, those who stay do not judge their sisters who choose this very difficult path of survival.

Throughout their years of captivity, the women find ways to keep themselves occupied, including using their voices to produce a choral orchestra, as they have no other instruments. This allows them a means by which to transcend their suffering, as they each focus on learning and performing their parts and contributing meaningfully to the choir so that each song succeeds. Functioning on one level simply as a compelling distraction from the adverse conditions, the orchestra also provides the women with an avenue to power. By this act of singing, they are refusing to be completely oppressed or to succumb to the camp's gross dehumanisation. As singers, each with their individual voice to contribute, all the women become part of a larger identity – an orchestra with a creative and beautiful purpose – rather than just another faceless, walking almost-corpse. They are thus engaged in an exercise of soft power – power that serves human needs and desires yet does not oppress (Nye, 2004). It also models a higher form of humanity – that which can create and sustain something meaningful from nothing – in stark contrast to the cruel and destructive approach exemplified by their captors.

While some die, and all face the reality that they may be doomed, the women do not give up on life. This fortitude is encapsulated in an important scene towards the end of the film in which the choir director, frail and dying, shares her final words of wisdom with her comrades, saying of their Japanese captors, "I can't hate them. The worse they behave, the sorrier I feel for them". This gives the group moral power and purpose, and the courage with which to enact this strength of purpose. This concept is also embedded in the film's title, *Paradise Road*, which refers to the inevitable journey towards death that everyone living is on. Along the way, this journey may be sublimely beautiful, terrifyingly horrendous and everything in between, but the journey itself – and its endpoint – is inescapable.

This story, although relating extreme experience and a dark period of history, highlights nurses growing into resilience and can be directly related to contemporary professional experience. Each of the nurses (and the other women) in this camp, in their own way, creatively responds to, and copes with, the adverse situation in which they find themselves. When there is no food, they find it. When there is no medicine, they obtain it by trading what they do have. In the face of violence, they enact non-violent resistance. When others attempt to dehumanise them, they actively reclaim their humanity. While they are not able to manage the adversity at its source (that is, by vanquishing their gaolers or physically escaping), nor do they simply passively accept their situation. Instead, they routinise the traumatic, developing daily schedules which they can control. They also turn their attention to productive actions, in effect suppressing the source of adversity. Routinising the traumatic lessens its emotional cadence and assists in making unbearable work (and other situations) more bearable (Chambliss, 1996). Such practices are often effective coping strategies for traumatic situations – something that unfortunately many nurses face in their careers. As discussed in an earlier chapter, a phenomenon associated with nursing stress is "second victimisation", which is where caregivers closely associated with a person undergoing a traumatic experience, actually suffer similarly and may find themselves with symptoms of post-traumatic stress (Seys et al., 2013). Thus, the more nurses prepare for such possibilities, the greater the likelihood they will have sufficient coping resources to enable them to remain resilient (Hegney et al., 2015).

More than machines

Nurses also have upcoming traumas to face. In thinking about the future, science fiction can present a vision for a better world, or warnings about it, especially if the audience takes note of the underlying messages (James, 2012). In the short film *Robo Nurse* (Usherwood, 2009), one possible future is imagined as society struggles to solve the ongoing crisis of nursing supply. Set in 2020, the ruling "Fascist Benevolent Neo-conservative Party" has created a prototype for the future of nursing, a fully robotic nurse. Managed by a technician, the robot fits onto a trolley and is fuelled by a nuclear power cell, making it cheap and clean to run. Modelled as a statuesque, strong-looking female, the robot nurse speaks in a mechanical, emotionless voice and moves slowly and somewhat clumsily, but assesses patients' medical conditions accurately and efficiently. Its main deficit is that it operates without any sense of empathy or human understanding. Threatening to make human nurses redundant, nurses protest this development. Their collectivisation is, however, quickly outlawed. This drives them underground and forces them into the position of resistance fighters, although their struggle seems doomed.

The animated cartoon, *Big Hero 6* (2014) presents a far more utopian view of robot nurses. In this representation, the robot is genderless and made from white, inflatable rubber. This nurse is not only able to perform instant assessments and effective treatments, but is also friendly, intuitive and empathic. Moreover, it is portable and when not needed, can be deflated and folded away into a discrete package.

Today, robotic science has made significant inroads in health care practices – making lifesaving surgeries more precise and safe (Boys et al., 2016). Robots are already assisting people with disabilities to communicate, move paralysed limbs, dress and eat, and affording those who are isolated the ability to access experts for diagnosis and treatment (Wang et al., 2017). Such robotic advances may, indeed, offer many advantages over human care giving. Robots do not get fatigued. Nor do they allow emotion to override logic or make human errors. They can also work in dangerous situations for unlimited periods. Yet, despite these advances in the practical use of robots, many of the ethical and other issues potentially involved in their use as nurses are raised and discussed in popular fiction rather that other fora. In Issac Asimov's classic collection of stories, *I, Robot* (1950), the first tale, "Robbie", first published in 1940, is set more than a half century into the future in late 1990s. Revised for the 1950 collection, the Robbie of the title is a robot, a nursemaid to Gloria, and the story focuses on Gloria's mother's anxieties about this new technology. Fearing her daughter has become too attached to a non-human machine, the mother returns Robbie to the factory. Gloria is inconsolable, and almost dies in the attempt to be reunited with her nurse. It is only when Robbie uses her robot abilities to save Gloria, that her mother is persuaded that robots can be trusted.

In emphasising and often magnifying and even pre-empting issues that society is ignoring, popular fiction can thus point to issues and advances to which people need to pay attention. Today, in association with, and in addition to, advances in, robotics, other technological solutions to health and health care issues are being avidly pursued, and richly funded, by govern-ments, businesses and private individuals. These include artificial intelligence, genetic engineering, nanotechnology and virtual reality. While these develop-ments bring the promise of new and more effective ways to understand, manage and prevent diseases and disorders (Meskó, 2014), they are also unset-tling, providing suggestive material for the imaginations of astute storytellers. In reality, robots are not (yet) capable of providing compassion and warmth, enabling patients to feel listened to and, as a result, fully cared for. In response to this point, Usherwood's film underscores the need for human beings to remain in control of patient care, understanding that nurses take a leadership role in humanely focused care, following Joseph Campbell, who stated that such humanity comes not from the machine, but from the heart (1988, p. 24).

Yet, as has been discussed in earlier chapters, there are times when nurses have not stepped up to this responsibility, and this has led to the dehumanisa-tion of patients, with devastating outcomes. It is thus a component of the nurse's role to ensure that the "human face" of care is emphasised – through valuing personal touch, connection and conversation, and being responsive to each patient's unique needs and strengths. Fictional narratives about robot nurses also serve as a reminder that despite its promise, there is a tension between the advances that technology can provide and humanistically-focused care. Some have argued that nurses need to take a role in negotiating and easing that tension, so that patients can accept the benefits of develop-ments in technology, and health care workers embrace new tools, without too much resistance (Barnard and Sandelowski, 2001; Salzmann-Erikson and Eriksson, 2016). To, however, take up this leadership role, nurses must be secure in their values and not, for instance, see themselves as subservient in the health care system. They must also not allow themselves to become absorbed in the mindless, repetitive completion of routine tasks. Empowered nurses, who are sure of their position within the health system, know that they perform critical roles of treatment provider, health educator, team member and leader, and are thus proactive in taking action to prevent distress or dysfunction.

Nurses knowing their value

An excerpt from the first series of *The Good Doctor* (episode 6, 2017) contains a vivid illustration of a nurse who has this confident knowledge of her value. The night shift is just beginning in the Emergency Department and three junior doctors are attending. Commenting on how quiet it is, they share a joke with Nurse Farrar (played by Kari Coleman). Smiling, Nurse Farrar then answers a ringing telephone. Her smile fades as she asks, "How long?" and then "Got it!". Hanging up, she immediately moves into action. Her voice switches in register and volume as she addresses her team directly. "Listen up everybody. We've got a mass cas coming in. Bus crash. Two dozen passengers. Transfer all patients waiting for beds up to the nursing units. Have maintenance bring down cots". She continues to explain, "We're going to convert the waiting room into triage. No one goes home until we're all clear". No words are wasted, no order is ambiguous. Her actions demonstrate how the nature of nursing requires that clinicians possess the ability to move from the mundane to the urgent in an instant. In this example, as in life, nurses cannot afford to be uncertain of their role or reserved in providing direction to a multi-disciplinary team.

Conclusion

It is often noted that nurses practice at important life transitions, or thresholds, where danger and change are imminent (Buchanan, 1997). These are challenging moments and resting in the shadows, giving purpose to a nurse's reassuring presence, are the values and moral purpose of the role that have developed through the realities of practice. *The Nun's Story, The English Patient and Paradise Road* all exemplify this strength of purpose as demonstrated by the nurse characters in these narratives. These emotionally charged stories of how suffering can lead to personal redemption and fulfillment reveal the potential of humanity, and how transcending injustice and staying focused on a higher purpose, can lead to social change. The stories also reveal a paradox that often confronts nurses: that sometimes a nurse can feel as though they have become a slave to the system that they are meant to be taking an active part in. There can be situations when they feel they have no choice but to comply with overriding and even oppressive policies, or when a nurse is denied the opportunity to work with patients in a proactive way. Nurses who know their value, however, who are aware they have a unique and complementary role to doctors and understand their importance in terms of being a member of a health care team, can be empowered professionals, not diffident or uncertain.

Buchanan (1997) argues that nurse characters in stories often play a donor role, in that they are helpers who facilitate progression in other characters. Nurse Hana in *The English Patient* is an example of this, but as the brief analysis of her actions and character has revealed, her role is much more than secondary. She also has her own hero's journey to undertake. Nurse Hana practices like other nurses in war, on the threshold of life and death; her participation in war is characterised by the awareness that, at any time, death can occur. Rules that work well in peacetime may not apply, and much of the work of nurses and doctors is narrowed down to be about facilitating the safe transition from soldier to patient, and back again. Within *The English Patient*, however, Hana's awakening and transformation occur because she bravely faces a patient in an abject state, and realises that she identifies with his alienation. Together, they each start to learn about life and living, she shares his epiphanies, and so she learns and changes. Hana's path is a lesson in humility and redemption.

A transformation in purpose and identity also comes about in *Paradise Road*. Instead of the women becoming self-focused, or the group disintegrating into cliques, they bond as a group. Despite the heartbreaking deaths of some of its members, the strength of shared purpose, empathy and support enables the group to adapt, endure and retain a sense of hope. Within this group, no single individual attempts to speak for everyone, or possesses the necessary qualities to steer the group politically, physically or emotionally the entire time. Instead, each person is shown to have unique strengths that are co-opted and put to use to foster the survival and wellbeing of the group. This distributes the burden and risk, at the same time also allowing each individual to find their niche and be of use for the good of the group. While some members are (or become) more vulnerable than others, the collective strength helps the group maintain hope and direction, and – in turn – provides a model of acting that can be internalised and personally owned by each individual. Women who may otherwise have given up, thus find the courage to endure. In this way, there is a clear reason to maintain one's membership. While these dark stories delve into the realities of adverse events faced by, and facing, nurses, they also highlight possibilities for transformation and professional growth. The social cohesion and the value of each individual's contribution to the collective that they emphasise are two important resilience strategies that are of use today in contemporary nursing.

Challenges facing nursing are many, including those forecast by the looming reality that some of nursing's work may be replaced through machine learning and robots. Representations in popular culture are assisting to raise such challenges for public discussion and contemplation.

References

Asimov I (1950) *I, Robot.* New York: Gnome Press.

Barnard A and Sandelowski M (2001) Technology and humane nursing care: (Ir)reconcilable or invented difference? *Journal of Advanced Nursing* 34(3): 367–375.

Beresford B (dir) (1997) *Paradise Road.* Film. Sydney: Samson productions.

Boys J, Alicuben E, Demeester M, Worrell S, Oh D, Hagen J and Demeester S (2016) Public perceptions on robotic surgery, hospitals with robots, and surgeons that use them *Surgical Endoscopy* 30(4): 1310–1316.

Buchanan T (1997) Nursing our narratives: Towards a dynamic understanding of a narrative simply as a transparent window opening onto new nurses in narrative tales *Nursing Inquiry* 4: 80–87.

Campbell J and Moyers B (1988) *The Power of Myth.* New York: Anchor.

Chambliss D F (1996) *Beyond Caring: Hospitals, Nurses, and the Social Organization of Ethics.* Chicago: University of Chicago Press.

Conti-O'Hare M (2002) *The Nurse as Wounded Healer: From Trauma to Transcendence.* New York: Jones and Bartlett.

Corso V (2012) Oncology nurse as wounded healer: Developing a compassion identity. *Clinical Journal of Oncology Nursing* 16(5): 448–450.

Dunn C (2000) *Wounded Healer of the Soul: An Illustrated Biography.* New York: Parabola Books.

Foucault M (2005) *Histoire de la folie à l'âge classique.* Paris: Edition Gallimard.

Hall J. (1997). Nurses as Wounded Healers. *The Australian Journal of Holistic Nursing* 4(1): 11–16.

Hall D and Williams C (dirs) (2014) *Big Hero 6*. Film. Hollywood: Walt Disney Pictures.

Haswell J and Edwards E (2004) *The English Patient* and his narrator: "Opener of the ways" *Studies in Canadian Literature* 29(2): 122–140.

Hegney D, Rees C, Eley S, Osseiran-Moisson R and Francis K (2015) The contribution of individual psychological resilience in determining the professional quality of life of Australian nurses *Frontiers in Psychology* 6: 1–8.

Heinrich K (1992) Create a tradition: Teach nurses to share stories. *Journal of Nursing Education* 31(3): 141–143.

Hulme K (dir) (1956) *The Nun's Story*. New York: Little, Brown.

James S (2012) *Maps of Utopia*. Oxford: Oxford University Press.

Jann M (dir) (2017) Not fake. *The Good Doctor* episode 6, series 1. Television series. Sony Pictures Television: San Jose.

Loomis R (1991) *The Grail: From Celtic myth to Christian Symbol*. Princeton: Princeton University Press.

Jeffrey B (1954) *White Coolies*. Sydney: Angus and Robertson.

McAllister M (2014) Vivian Bullwinkel: A model of resilience and a symbol of strength *Collegian* 22: 135–141.

McAllister M (2017) Nurse as wounded healer in *The English Patient*. *TEXT* special issue 38. Available at: www.textjournal.com.au/speciss/issue38/content.htm.

Meskó B (2014) Disruption: Technology trends in medicine and health care *The Futurist* May–June: 31–38.

Minghella A (dir) (1996) *The English Patient*. Film. Hollywood: Miramax.

Nelson S (2010) *Say Little, Do Much: Nursing, Nuns, and Hospitals in the Nineteenth Century*. Philadelphia: University of Pennsylvania Press.

Nunan D (2011) Fault lines: Scars as text in Michael Ondaatje's *The English Patient* and *Anil's Ghost*. *University of Alberta Health Sciences Journal* 6(1): 14–16.

Nye J (2004) *Soft Power: The Means to Success in World Politics*. London: Hachette.

Ondaatje M (1993) *The English Patient*. New York: Vintage Books.

Paul E (1985) Wounded healers: A summary of the Vietnam nurse veteran project *Military Medicine* 150(11): 571–576.

Salzmann-Erikson M and Eriksson H (2016) Tech-resistance: The complexity of implementing nursing robots in healthcare workplaces *Contemporary Nurse* 52(5): 567–568.

Seys D, Wu A, Gerven E, Vleugels A, Euwema M, Panella M and Vanhaecht K (2013) Health care professionals as second victims after adverse events: A systematic review *Evaluation and the Health Professions* 36(2): 135–162.

Sharp S, McAllister M and Broadbent M (2015) The vital blend of clinical competence and compassion: How patients experience person-centred care. *Contemporary Nurse* 52(2–3): 1–13.

Traynor M and Evans A (2014) Slavery and jouissance: analysing complaints of suffering in UK and Australian nurses' talk about their work. *Nursing Philosophy* 15(3): 192–200.

Usherwood F (2009) *Robo Nurse*. [Short film]. Winner of the Geneva Labour Film Shorts. Retrieved from Festivalwww.youtube.com/watch?v=DAB6eGzOnIs

Wang R, Sudhama A, Begum M, Huq R and Mihailidis A (2017) Robots to assist daily activities: Views of older adults with Alzheimer's disease and their caregivers *International Psychogeriatrics* 29(1): 67–79.

Zinnemann F (dir) (1959) *The Nun's Story*. Film. Hollywood: Warner Brothers.

Conclusion
Out of the shadows, into the light

Storytelling is a prominent way that humans communicate and convey ideas, beliefs and customs to each other (Bruner, 2010). Recently, public storytelling has been enjoying a resurgence, as its power to convey information in a memorable form, emotionally activate listeners and aid in building connections between them, has found new outlets in podcasts, online libraries and live events (LeBlanc, 2017). As such, storytelling has long been a part of nursing's culture (Wolf, 1986). The aim of this book has not been to define or describe the wide range of stereotypes that exist about nurses and nursing in such narratives. This has been done ably and comprehensively by others (see, for instance, Kalisch and Kalisch, 1987; Summers and Summers, 2015). Nor has the purpose of the book been to make judgements about whether such stereotypical representations serve a useful and worthwhile or hurtful or destructive purpose. Rather, this book has discussed how tropes of the figure of the nurse, which are shorthand ways of representing nursing, feature across a range of narratives and how this imagery makes stories compelling. This focus is built on the premise that the narratives disseminated through popular culture are influential, and not insignificant. We have also written with a readership in mind that includes both nurses and non-nurses – such as scholars of popular culture and social scientists.

Our initial interest in the topic of the dark side of nursing's image, was spurred by the realisation of how vividly figures such as Nurse Ratched have endured in public consciousness and what this might mean for nursing. In our analysis, we propose that the examination of the shadow side of nursing – that is, the dimension of nursing that is not motherly or angelic, sacred or self-sacrificing but is, instead, flawed, impatient, ambivalent or nefarious – is important because it is just as much a part of nursing as the virtuous aspects of the profession. We drew from Jung's belief that we all have a shadow side, parts of our personality that we may repress or push outside of conscious awareness because they are painful, shameful or even repulsive. We were also inspired by how individuals may be able to turn to this hidden side of themselves, to become more self-aware. So too, can groups and professions appreciate a propensity for complexity and contradiction. In terms of nursing, this is important, for this understanding may illuminate such perplexing issues as how it is that individuals can start out as caring and compassionate but slip into actions such as patient neglect, bullying, coverups, and even outright crime.

In this book, we have therefore looked to a range of representations of the shadow side of nurses and nursing in popular culture in order to begin to make sense of these conundrums. Medical dramas proliferate on television and in film and nurses, being the largest workforce in health, are of course a familiar feature of these productions. Mostly, nursing roles on screen are benign, and are included simply to provide aesthetic or romantic interest. Significant dramatic action is more frequently left to the medicos who problem solve, and either make serious errors and be called to account, or be exalted for their brilliance. Occasionally, however, nurses are cast as more major characters. When these nursing characters are malevolent, dangerous or out of control, some of these storylines are so arresting that they become seared into popular memory.

Characterisations and storylines can also illuminate other anxieties around nurses and nursing which are rarely voiced. This can be seen in representations of nurses barely coping – as seen in the television series *Nurse Jackie* or described in contemporary memoirs by nurses, or where nurses are insidious collaborators in murder. This imaging reveals how nurses hold real and great power over the vulnerable and, if they wish, can act as assassins as well as saviours.

Imagery of nurses acting in unrestrained, unethical ways is disconcerting. But when such behaviour is hidden, covered up or the individual constructed as a monstrous anomaly, as it is in *Dirty John* or *The Good Nurse*, a greater damage can occur. If those in charge of health services, and ultimately society, do not consider their own part in enabling neglect or corruption to occur, then the risk of future damage continues. While evil nurses make for compelling and entertaining storytelling, they are worth considering more deeply, for deliberately neglecting, hurting or killing patients are not simply the heinous acts of aberrant individuals. They can be signs of a health care system that does not respond quickly enough to wrongdoing. The system may have been left to operate too long without public scrutiny or standards checked, and toxic professional cultures may have developed. Shining a light on this dark underbelly of health care can, therefore, provide a first step towards identifying the complex factors that cause systemic problems and guide constructive remedial action. Thinking about, and then analysing, popular narratives about nurses in this way offers an opportunity to prompt reflection upon nursing work and its place in the world. This analysis also considers why people see nurses in the ways they do.

The shadow side

Carl Jung considered that human beings are complex, with a personality that is made up of that which is consciously projected – our persona, which is what we would like others to see – and a hidden side to our self which is repressed into the unconscious. Jung referred to this as the "shadow", both because it is hidden and because it consists of primitive, negative or socially disparaged emotions like lust, anger and shame. Obscured from consciousness, this part of the personality is unenlightened and dark. Yet, like all objects' shadows, it is also ever-present, connected to the self, influencing behaviour and contributing to the whole. In Jung's (1938) words, "everyone carries a shadow, and the less it is embodied in the individual's conscious life, the blacker and denser it is" (p. 131). There are many stories about nursing in popular culture that, when closely examined, reveal this insight. Stories about nurses who are fallen angels, for instance, Cath Hardacre in *Trust Me* and Edith Kiefer in *Fog in August*, provide vital lessons for nurses if sustained engagement with these texts is fostered.

Mythic stories about past and present, good and evil, and life and death, can resonate deeply with those who reflect upon them. *The English Patient*, for example, can be read as simply a tale about a dying man reflecting on his life. As we have shown, however, the story can also be interpreted more imaginatively, as a parable about wounded healers, and about an individual's propensity for taking right or wrong actions. As Joseph Campbell writes, one of the greatest lessons for humans is to realise that "heaven and hell are within us" (Campbell and Moyers, 2011, p. 46). This is why enduringly popular narratives such as *One Flew Over the Cuckoo's Nest* and *Misery*, do not only have value as highly entertaining creative works. They can also prompt reflection on values, and even ultimately clarify them – in the process offering direction for nurses. Nurses, although many are motivated by their desire to care for others, undeniably exist in a powerful position in relation to vulnerable patients, and thus there needs to be checks within the health care system to ensure that wrongdoing – whether caused by error or intent – is prevented or corrected.

As Jungian analysts explain, the negative proclivities that we all possess tend to be repressed and can be projected onto unwitting adversaries. Unfortunately, all too frequently, there are reports of this occurring in health care contexts, with nurses projecting their own anxieties onto others. Patients can bear the brunt of nursing stress and be subjected to neglect or dehumanisation (Haque and Waytz, 2012). This projection can also manifest as lateral violence directed towards other nurses (Roberts, 2015) or doctors being unfairly disparaged by nurses (Fagin and Garelick, 2004). These effects are some of the skeletons in nursing's closet that, although seemingly difficult to address in professional arenas, are referenced in both mainstream contemporary fictions such as *Nurse Jackie* and *Getting On*, as well as in historical dramas. There are yet darker issues affecting nursing, such as the risk of patient abuse and even willful murder. These situations, fraught with tension and drama, can provide rich material for storytellers but are also important aspects of nursing's culture that need to be scrutinised. *Fog in August*, *Dirty John* and *The Good Nurse* are recent examples of narratives in popular culture which have awakened at least some to the reality that not all health professionals have benevolent intent, and why the highest standards of both professional practice and regulation are essential in health care.

This is not to assert that popular culture satisfactorily conveys the complexities of the reality of nursing to its consumers – or that it has ever had the intention of doing so. Popular culture is not a preferred source to access the technical facts and details of nursing. Nor should it be, as this is not the function of popular culture. What popular culture can do, and sometimes does extremely well, is to cast a light on the underlying issues and paradoxes that interest, challenge or perplex society. Because narratives are polysemic, with many meanings that are individually determined by their consumers, not everyone will notice subtexts, or make the same meaning from them.

In the sustained readings presented in this book, we have identified and discussed several core ideas. First, there remains an unresolved cultural anxiety towards institutions such as health care, which can be seen to exert power and control over patients and staff. This is a theme that runs through many hospital thrillers such as *The Ward* and *Fragile* as well as dark comedies such as *Getting On*. In such representations, the activities, emotions, doubts and fears of nurses that are normally concealed from the public are displayed. Rather than operating smoothly and efficiently, these stories portray disturbances to health services that can intensify or confirm audiences' trepidations. Such narratives are compelling because they reflect how society continues to have concerns about health care systems and authority figures. This anxiety relates to the influence and direction that medical science has over our lives. It also points to a concern that most individuals have only limited input into, or knowledge about, how to regulate and enforce the necessary practical, ethical and moral safeguards.

In such narratives, nurses are also acknowledged as powerful, but this power can be feared. The ongoing response to films such as *Misery* and the outcry over the proposed Netflix series *Ratched* are examples of this. A nurse's access to knowledge, power and the tools for change play an important role in the plotting of such narratives. Yet there is a paradox inherent in this positioning. Nurses are endowed with power. However, at the same time this power can be corrupting.

The gendered nature of nursing is an integral part of nursing's historical and contemporary identity, as well as the source of a number of problems with which it has struggled. That nurses find both pride and shame in their gendered identity and achievements, is an important paradox evident in some representations of nursing in popular culture. Femininity can be imaged as a strength or a weakness in popular culture, a complexity that creates tensions when nursing is represented in this way. The enduring trope of the good nurse is closely linked to an outdated feminine ideal, exemplified in the image of *Betty Boop*. The good nurse is an attractive and amenable woman who is caring, selfless and non-threatening. Such a stereotype is romantic and nostalgic for many nurses as well as patients, but it is also limiting, silencing and sexist. Furthermore, it has become so entrenched and commonplace that, even for nursing students, the script for how to embody the role of a nurse comes already pre-packaged and is difficult to rewrite. The reality of nursing work requires very different attributes and skills than what were espoused two centuries ago. Thus, these narratives need to be decoded with a critical stance, or at least with an appreciation for how they cast an image of nursing that no longer holds in practice.

The attractive, desirable, sexy nurse is another often-repeated trope that is a derivation of the good nurse stereotype. In this image, ideals of femininity and desirability are emphasised, although not, of course, demureness. At the same time, strength, allure and influence are also evoked. Exemplified by Margaret "Hot Lips" Houlihan, the sexy nurse is captivating, provocative and difficult to ignore. In most stories, this imaging of the sexy nurse is demeaning, but she/he is also eye-catching. This trope is interesting because it draws on the paradox that the public can see nurses as simultaneously proper and extremely improper. Fagin and Diers (1983) theorised that this contradiction rests in an unresolved anxiety held about intimacy and the body. Reactions to the undressed body in the context of a sexual relationship are certainly very different to reactions to that same naked body in the context of medical procedures and nursing actions. But there may be subtle overlaps in the human emotions engendered including feelings of embarrassment, shame or desire. Imaging the nurse as sexually attractive links the profession to desire, need and appeal. It also makes nursing distinctive and visible. These positive aspects have been recently co-opted by innovative public health initiatives to encourage health service utilisation. Time will tell if the image of the sexy nurse can continue to be reclaimed in ways that are effective and empowering.

Although nursing is no longer a career exclusively for women, it remains a challenge to recruit men to nursing and to create gender balance (Clow, Ricciardelli and Bartfay, 2015). The films *Magnolia* and *Chronic* are unusual for a number of reasons, not least because they feature in-depth studies of nursing in action but also as that work is performed by male nurses. Gender is not, however, the focus of this storytelling. These nurses have intriguing personalities and backstories and, furthermore, their nursing work is atypical, as it is home-based (not in a hospital) and autonomous (rather than team-work). Patients in their care are assisted to die peacefully, and these nurses work with them skillfully and compassionately, thus revealing the complexity of nursing work. Nursing is depicted as technical, although sometimes tedious, emotionally challenging and, sometimes, as a profession where the needed support is not forthcoming.

These films also exemplify a rarely discussed dimension of nursing. This is its class-based positioning. Nursing is a profession that is, for many, firmly working class (Connell, 2010). This is yet another paradox that contributes to nursing identity, for despite the importance of nursing to society, its contribution is not valued highly in economic terms. Nurses are depicted as accepting inhospitable working hours and conditions and tolerating hostility from others in order to secure a decent income. These depictions expose some of the realities of the ongoing struggle of the working class. *Nurse Jackie, Getting On* and *Trust Me* also detail the negative consequences of declining conditions for a profession that once held the promise of an elevated status for its graduates. Jackie steals restricted drugs to control the symptoms of a back injury that would otherwise put her out of work and propel her family into poverty. Kim Wilde must absorb humiliation without protest because she has no authority within the hierarchy and Cath Hardacre takes another desperate route. After having her character impugned, career destroyed and her family's sole income taken away, she resorts to identity theft and weaves a tangled web of imposture and deceit. This threatens the lives of patients and her own freedom.

Moving into the light

According to Jungian philosophy, accepting the shadow side involves individuals in the acknowledgement that negative and painful emotions, failure, inadequacy and evil exists – or has potential to exist – inside themselves, just as much as it does in any other person (Jung, 1969; Watts, 1961). Acknowledging and accepting their own shadow side makes a person stronger, more whole. This is described as integration, the achievement of a sense of unity with the result of an absence of conflict in one's own identity. Awareness of the shadow side of the self is not about the elimination of feelings such as anxiety but acceptance of their existence, without resort to self-recrimination. Acknowledgement of negative parts also allows the positives to be appreciated. Furthermore, this acceptance of good and evil in one's own self leads to an awareness of the shadow side in others. In the context of health care, this can lead to accepting difficult realities. As Jung (2001) stated:

> It is a moral achievement on the part of the doctor who ought not to let himself [sic] be repelled by sickness and corruption. We cannot change anything unless we accept it. Condemnation does not liberate, it oppresses. If the doctor wishes to help a human being, he must be able to accept him as he is. And he can do this in reality only when he has already seen and accepted himself as he is.
>
> (p. 240)

He also admitted how challenging this can be, adding, "this sounds simple, but simple things are always the most difficult" (p. 240).

These insights have a number of important implications that are directly applicable to nursing. The first insight is that being aware of propensity for evil can protect one from being hurt. In nursing, this may mean that the expectation of adversity can be protective. It is well known that nursing is a stressful profession where secondary trauma, witnessing the adversity of others, can be very damaging (Seys et al., 2013), and nursing scholars argue that students need to be prepared for this impending reality (Hanson and McAllister, 2017). The second insight is that when unhappiness or bitterness first arises at work, it needs to be declared, not avoided or repressed. Many workplaces become toxic because those working in them do not speak up soon enough (Croft and Cash, 2012). Not only does such openness allow an individual to practice self-care, but it contributes to an overall climate of honesty and authentic communication that can offer the possibility for others and the system to self-correct.

The third insight is that the knowledge that one is capable of harm can be a motivator to be much more cautious and careful in one's actions. For Peterson (2002), this is the meaning of being virtuous. That is, virtue is not about being harmless and therefore impotent or passive. Instead, it is about knowing one has power but choosing not to harm. Fourth, significant learning can take place when one voluntarily makes contact with that which frightens or disgusts. This is a hallmark of Jungian psychoanalytic theory – "In sterquiliniis invenitur" which, translated from Latin, means "In filth it will be found" (Peterson, 2002, p. 44). This means that in both the world and the unconscious mind, there are difficult aspects of life or being that disappoint or disgust. When they are avoided and repressed, one is left undeveloped. But acknowledging and facing these challenging parts of being human can make a person stronger. For this reason, the abject experiences that are common in nursing, yet rarely discussed at length, need to be brought into the open. Such difficult and negative encounters make the nursing identity more whole, and with open discussion, mean that nurses can be better prepared for challenging encounters and more fully armed with coping skills.

Many of the nursing characters discussed in this book – Ratched, Kiefer, Wilkes, Hardacre and others – were caught in the negative powers of an abyss. We cannot know what might have happened if they had faced their demons, but perhaps they would have been able to change the ending of their stories, take heroic action, resolve their own anxieties and change the world for others.

References

Bruner J (2010) Narrative, culture, and mind. In Schiffrin D, de Fina A and Nylund A (eds) *Telling Stories: Language, Narrative, and Social Life*. Washington: Georgetown University Press, 45–49.

Campbell J and Moyers B (2011) *The Power of Myth*. New York: Anchor.

Clow K, Ricciardelli R and Bartfay W (2015) Are you man enough to be a nurse? The impact of ambivalent sexism and role congruity on perceptions of men and women in nursing advertisements. *Sex Roles* 72(7–8): 363–376.

Connell J (2010) *Migration and the Globalisation of Health Care: The Health Worker Exodus?* Cheltenham: Edward Elgar Publishing.

Croft R and Cash P (2012) Deconstructing contributing factors to bullying and lateral violence in nursing using a postcolonial feminist lens. *Contemporary Nurse* 42(2): 226–242.

Fagin L and Diers D (1983) Nursing as metaphor. *New England Journal of Medicine* 309: 116–117.

Fagin L and Garelick A (2004) The doctor-nurse relationship. *Advances in Psychiatric Treatment* 10(4): 277–286.

Hanson J and McAllister M (2017) Preparing for workplace adversity: Student narratives as a stimulus for learning. *Nurse Education in Practice* 25: 89–95.

Haque O and Waytz A (2012) Dehumanization in medicine: Causes, solutions, and functions. *Perspectives on Psychological Science* 7(2): 176–186.

Jung CG (1938) Psychology and religion. In *Collected Works, Vol. 11: Psychology and Religion: West and East*. London: Pantheon.

Jung C (1969) *Archetypes and the Collective Unconscious. Collected Works of C.G. Jung, Volume 9 (Part 1)*. Princeton: Princeton University Press.

Jung C (2001) *Modern Man in Search of a Soul*. Abingdon: Taylor & Francis.

Kalisch P and Kalisch B (1987) *The Changing Image of the Nurse*. Menlo-Park: Addison-Wesley.

LeBlanc R (2017) Digital story telling in social justice nursing education *Public Health Nursing* 34(4): 395–400.

Peterson J (2002) *Maps of Meaning: The Architecture of Belief*. New York: Routledge.

Roberts S (2015) Lateral violence in nursing: A review of the past three decades *Nursing Science Quarterly* 28(1): 36–41.

Seys D, Wu A, Gerven E, Vleugels A, Euwema M, Panella M and Vanhaecht K (2013) Health care professionals as second victims after adverse events: A systematic review. *Evaluation & The Health Professions* 36(2): 135–162.

Summers S and Summers H (2015) *Saving Lives: Why the Media's Portrayal of Nursing Puts Us All at Risk*. New York: Oxford University Press.

Watts A (1961) *Psychotherapy East and West*. London: Pantheon Books.

Wolf Z (1986) *Nursing Rituals in an Adult Acute Care Hospital: An Ethnography*. Dissertation. Philadelphia: University of Pennsylvania.

Index

Abaan, S 34
Abeni, M 75
abjection 5, 65–80, 155, 164
adversity, coping with 146–157,
    163–164
aesthetics 38–39, 42, 57, 159
aged care 20, 109
ageing 21
agency, nurses' own 25, 42
Agrillo, C 87
Aiken, L 102
Akin, Joseph Dewey 122
Alavi, C 140
Alberti, J 18
Alchin, S 140
All Saints (Lee, 1998–2009) 65
Allan, H 66
Allitt, Beverley 122, 124–125
alter-egos 123
altruism 1, 23, 97, 148
Anderson, Paul Thomas 72, 73, 75
Anderson, Peggy 98
Andrews, J 142
Angel of Death (Proctor, 2005) 125
Angelo, Richard 122, 124
angels: angel of mercy 7, 74; angels of
    death 74, 121–126; nurses as angels 3,
    9, 10, 52, 71, 100
anxiety: acceptance of shadow side 163,
    164; cultural anxiety 74, 87, 159, 161;
    as form of mental illness 140; ghost
    stories 90–91; irresolvable anxieties 23;
    and the monstrous nurse 103; nurses' 6,
    23, 72, 90, 91–92, 134, 160; patients' 5,
    51, 66, 74, 89, 91, 104, 110, 150;
    projection of 7, 51, 60, 160;
    unconscious 57
Anzac Girls (ABC, 2014) 9
apparitions 83–85

appearance (physical) 2, 9, 52, 100, 103;
    see also attractiveness; sexy nurse trope;
    uniforms
apprentice models 44
Archer, C 3
archetypes 7, 55–56, 58, 60, 97, 148–150
arts of nursing/medicine 35, 36, 38, 41
Ashforth, B 27
Asimov, Isaac 153
Askill, J 122, 125
asylums 83–84, 103–108, 136–139,
    140, 146
Atonement (McEwan, 2001) 1, 4, 9, 10, 18
attractiveness 9, 52–55, 60, 61, 100, 103
attrition rates in the profession 5, 102, 108
Augustine, Saint 24
austerity 3, 25
Austgard, K 39
Australia 139–142
authority, a nurse's 38, 52, 122, 161, 162
autonomous decision-making 20, 121
awe inspiring, nursing is 23

Bachrach, L 136
backgrounds, nurses' personal 26–27
bad/evil nurses 2–3, 97–113, 114–129
Bakhtin, M. 11
Balaguero, Jaume 89, 99
balance, achieving for patient 39
Barber, J 58
Barboza, D 54
Barnard, A 154
Barton, W 137
battleaxe imagery: *Cloud Atlas* (Mitchell,
    2004 Wachowski, Tykwer and
    Wachowski, 2012) 101; as common
    stereotype 7, 99–100; *Getting On*
    (BBC, 2009–2011) 22; *Nurse Jackie*
    (Brixius, Dunsky and Wallem,

2009–2015) 25; *One Flew Over the Cuckoo's Nest* (Forman, 1975) 103, 104; paradox of 10; in transgressive texts 97
Battles, E 77
Bayley, Sandy 82–83
Beardshaw, V 142
Beck, C 91
Bednarek, M. 23, 30
Beebe, D 86
being in the world 68–69
Bellas, M 27
Benedict, S 5, 116, 117, 120, 121
Benner, P 47, 86
Bennett, A 88
Beresford, Bruce 150
Berman, J 72
Bern-Klug, M 83
Betters, R 87
Betty, L 87
Betty Boop 54–55, 65, 161–162
Big Hero 6 (2014) 153
Billings, Adelaide 88
biotechnology 41
black comedy 4, 23–25
Blair, P 22
blogs 87
Bloom, S 107
bodily fluids/secretions 5, 19, 66, 71; *see also* abjection; disgust
body, mind and spirit balance 39
Bogner, M 125
Bogossian, F 110
Books, C 86
boring, nursing is often 28, 29
Bosanquet, A 85
Boston, P 75
boundaries, nursing transgresses 5–6
boundaries, professional 46
Bowen, M 90
Boys, J 153
Bradbury-Jones, C 71
Brajtman, S 90
Braun, M 90
Brayne, S 86, 87
Brien, D L 5, 6, 30, 59, 71, 74, 75, 86, 88, 90, 91
Briggs, J 87
Briggs, R 34
Broadbent, M 150
Brooks, I 86
Brotheridge, C 27
Brown, L 20
Brown, R 86

Bruner, J 158
Bryce, J 61
Buchanan, D 22
Buchanan, T 54, 59, 155
bullying cultures 22–23, 25
Burke, R 99
Burleigh, M 118, 119
burnout 27, 131
Butler, M 142
buxomness 22, 54, 58, 100

Call the Midwife (Thomas, 2012–current) 36, 40–42
callings/vocations 25, 82, 146, 147
Campbell, J 154, 160
capital punishment 75
career structures 102
Carlile, M 35
Carpenter, J 109
Carper, B 37, 38, 46
Carrier, J 136
Carry On Again Doctor (Thomas, 1969) 52
Carry on Doctor (Thomas, 1967) 51, 52, 100
Carry On Matron (Thomas, 1972) 52
Carry On Nurse (Thomas, 1959) 52, 99–100
Carter, H 140, 141
Carter, M 89
Carter, T 75
cartoons 52–53, 54
Cash, P 164
catharsis 90–92
Chambers, Kristy 25–29, 30
Chambliss, D F 152
change agents, nurses as 143, 155
chaos 26, 27, 57, 70, 84, 89, 104
Chapman, J 52, 109
Charon, R 36
Chelouche, T 117
Cheng, C 27
Chiron 148
Cho, E 86
Chojnacka, I 2, 58
Chow, W 136
Chronic (Franco, 2015) 72, 73, 75, 77–78, 162
Clarke, J 3
Clarke, R 107
class divisions 2, 21, 22, 162; *see also* working classes
cleanliness 58, 68–69, 71
Cleary, M 85

cleavage 54, 58; *see also* buxomness
climate disasters 75–77
clinical judgement skills 47
clinical placements 28
Clooney, N 138
Cloud Atlas (Mitchell, 2004 Wachowski, Tykwer and Wachowski, 2012) 59, 100–101
Clow, K 162
Cogdell, C 117
cognitive work 23, 29
Cohen, T 20
Colla, R 124
colleagues: conflict with 134; peer support 77, 86, 87, 151; team work 45, 151, 155; working with 21, 23, 24, 28, 45, 47, 87–88, 151, 156
collective identity 8
collective redemption 150–151, 156
collective unconscious 7, 115
comedy 51, 52, 99–100, 136, 161
compassion 1, 10, 19, 23, 41, 148, 149
computer games 59
con-artists 108, 122
conflict 134
connections with patients 41, 74, 154
Connell, J 162
context, nursing with a 37, 38
Conti-O'Hare, M 27, 148
Coombs, M 92
Corbin, J 106
corporatisation 29
Corr, C 72
corruption 115, 124, 131, 136, 159, 161, 163
Corso, V 150
cosplay 59
Cote, J E 8
counter-narratives 11, 30, 110
courage 38, 40, 47
Cowling III, W 90
Crandall, C 107
Creed, B 97, 101
crime genre 5; *see also* true crime
Crimson Field (Clark, Evans and O'Sullivan, 2014) 9, 99
critical incidents 19
critical thinking 42–44, 48
Croft, R 164
crone figures 88
Crowther, A 117, 118, 125
Cullen, Charles 122–124
culture, definition of 11

culture clashes 44
Cunningham, A 108
Currell, S 117
Curtis, V 75
Cuthbert, A 40

Danvers State Asylum 83–84
Darbyshire, P 2, 10, 22, 52, 57, 104, 106
Dark Knight, The (Nolan, 2008) 59
dark side of nursing 4–7, 34–50, 115, 126, 142, 158–163
Davies, H 6
Davies, N 125
Davis, C 74, 102
Dawson, A 90, 101–102
De Maria, W 141–142
Dean, Roger 122
death, dealing with 19, 45, 72–78, 82–83, 86–87, 90, 162; *see also* dying patients; laying out; palliative care
Death cafés 72
death row, working on 5
deep acting 27–28
dehumanisation 4, 7, 28, 59, 68, 110, 119, 126, 151, 153, 154, 160
Deichmann, R 77
déjà vu 4
DeLamotte, E 66
depression 26, 140
Dernley, S 75
desensitisation 134
desirability 60, 61, 162; *see also* attractiveness; sexy nurse trope
detention centres 5
devaluation of care 109–110
Dibdin, E 108
Dickens, Charles 67–68, 69
Diers, D 55, 162
Dirty John podcast 108
Dirty John: The Dirty Truth (Mast, 2019) 108, 159, 160–161
disability 5, 17, 117, 119, 153
discrimination 58
disengagement 21, 27, 136, 148
disgust 23, 66, 70, 71, 72, 75, 164
doctors: conflict with 43; ethical knowledge 41–42; *Getting On* (BBC, 2009–2011) 20, 21; narrative medicine 36; and nurses' own agency 42; as social elite 35; in TV dramas 159; witchcraft 34, 35; working with 30, 84, 160
documentaries 122, 138, 139
domestic responsibilities 106, 135

dominant ideologies, changing 17, 30, 52
Donahue, M 35, 38
Donahue, P 82
Donelan, K 34
Donnelly, Helene 131
Dossey, B M 39
Double, O 56
double-entendres 52, 54
Doyle, K 66
dreams 91
drug addiction 24, 108–109
Duffield, C M 5
Dunn, C 148
dying patients 19, 35, 46–47, 72–75, 86–87, 162; *see also* death, dealing with

economic rationalism 106, 124
education 36, 106, 109, 131; *see also* training
Edwards, E 150
Edwards, S 38
Edwards-Jones, Imogen 57
Egenes, K 66
Ehenreich, B 34, 35
Eisenstaedt, Alfred 60
elderly patients 20, 109
Eley, D 26
Elkind, P 124
Ellard, J 140
Ellis, K 17
embodied ways of being 4
emergency/disaster situations 76
emotional intelligence 47
emotional labour 27, 27–28, 29, 30, 38, 47, 70–71, 90, 164
empathy: central to modern nursing identity 2, 47–48; and dehumanisation 119; *English Patient, The* (Ondaatje, 1993 Minghella, 1996) 149; ethical knowledge 40, 42; fear of death 90; *Get Well Soon! My (Un)Brilliant Career as a Nurse* (Chambers, 2012) 27; *Getting On* (BBC, 2009–2011) 20, 23; *Nurse Jackie* (Brixius, Dunsky and Wallem, 2009–2015) 25; *Nurse's Story, A* (Shalof, 2005) 46; nursing as a fine art 38, 39; robotic nurses 153
empirical knowledge 38, 41, 42, 46, 47, 92
end-of-life issues 72; *see also* dying patients; palliative care
English, D 34, 35

English Patient, The (Ondaatje, 1993 Minghella, 1996) 147–149, 155, 160
Enlightenment 34
equality policies 20
ER (2003–2011) 58
Eriksson, H 154
Eriksson, K 38
Eriksson, U 102–103
eroticisation 57–59
ethical dilemmas 117–118
ethical knowledge 38, 40–42
ethical principles 121, 126, 133
eugenics 115, 117–119
euthanasia 74, 77, 117, 118–119, 120
Evan, M 132
Evans, A 71, 72, 134, 146
everyday, exploring the 51, 73
evidence-based practice 4, 44, 82, 85
exhausting, nursing is often 29, 70, 76
experiential knowledge 8, 35, 37, 42, 44, 46
"exposés" 57

Fagin, C 7, 55, 160, 162
Faludi, S 106
family-friendly, nursing is not 135
fatigue 6
fear: abjection 70, 71, 75, 77; of the battleaxe 100; of the dark 89; of death 90; fears revealed 90; at the hands of unkind nurses 102; hauntings 84; patients' 5, 6, 51; wartime 57; of women's strength and power 97, 99
"feeling states" 38
feelings, repression of nurses' own *see* emotional labour
Feldman, D 107
Felicie, Jacoba (Jacqueline Felice de Almania) 34–35
femininity 2, 55–56, 60, 161–162
feminism 30, 98–99, 104, 106, 109, 110
Fenwick, P 87
Ferns, T 2, 58
fetishisation of nursing 56, 57–59
Fida, R 134
Field, J 5, 122
filth/dirt, nurses must deal with 66
fine art of nursing 38
Fink, S 5, 76–77
First World War 69–70, 117
Fisher King 148
Fiske, J 17
flawed individuals 25

Fledderus, B 148
Fleisher, Max 54, 65
flippancy 21
Fog in August (Wessel, 2016) 114–121, 126, 160–161
folk-wisdom 34, 35
footwear 21, 58
Forman, M 103
Forsberg, A 102
Foster, J 125
Foster, R 85
Foth, T 120
Foucault, M 147
Fragile (Balaguero, 2005) 89, 91, 99, 161
Francis, R 48, 131, 142
Franco, Michael 72, 73–74, 75
Frank, A W 6
French, R 6
Freud, S 13, 56–57, 91
Frow, J 140
full moon superstitions 85
Fuller-Torrey, E 118
functional attitudes to nursing 21
funding climates 3, 24, 25, 131–132, 134, 137
funerals 83

Gadamer, H 38–39
gallows humour 77
game-playing 21
Gamp, Nurse Sairey 67–68, 69, 78
Garcez, A 87
Garelick, A 7, 160
Gecas, V 7
Geen, Benjamin 122
gender: and emotional labour 27; female identity and nursing 21; and fetishisation of nursing 59; and the history of nursing 146; inequality 106; male nurses 9, 21, 22, 34, 72–75, 97, 106, 123, 162; and mental illness 138; monstrous-feminine 97; Nurse Ratched 103–104; nursing as a gendered profession 2, 3, 30, 59, 60, 97–98, 106, 161–162
General Hospital (1963–current) 59
genocide 114–115, 119
Gerrard, S 52
Get Well Soon! My (Un)Brilliant Career as a Nurse (Chambers, 2012) 25–29, 30
Getting On (BBC, 2009–2011) 18–23, 29, 30, 99, 160, 161, 163

ghosts 4, 83–85, 86, 87–88, 89–90, 91, 92
Gillan, P 72
Gillespie, R 22
Giroux, H 11
Gittelman, M 115
glamorisation 23, 52
Godden, J 2
goddess myths 60
Goffard, Christopher 108
Goffman, Erving 138
Gonzalez, J 24
Good Doctor, The (2017) 41, 154–155
Good Nurse: A True Story of Medicine Madness and Murder (Graeber, 2014) 122–123, 159, 160–161
good nurse trope: battleaxe image subverts 100; *Carry On* films 52; and the complexities of caring 109; *Get Well Soon! My (Un)Brilliant Career as a Nurse* (Chambers, 2012) 27; *Getting On* (BBC, 2009–2011) 18, 21; history of 8–9; in Nazi Germany 117; *Nurse Jackie* (Brixius, Dunsky and Wallem, 2009–2015) 23–24; *Nurse's Story, A* (Shalof, 2005) 46; and nurses who kill 126; *Outlander* (Moore, 2014–current) 37; transgressions of 18, 97, 100; in TV dramas generally 17
good woman trope 8–9
Gordon, S 9, 10, 22, 46, 57, 97
Gorman, M 20
Gosport Independent Panel 142
Gothic 88, 91, 102
Gottschall, J 68
Gough, A 88
Gough, P 132
Gouthro, T 84
Graeber, C (*Good Nurse*) 5, 122–124, 159, 160–161
Grafton, Sue 98
Grandey, A 27
Gray, B 28, 115
Gray, F 53
Greek mythology 56, 60, 148
Green, M 35
Grice-Swenson, D 91
grief, dealing with 41, 75
Griffiths, J 55
Griffiths, P 106
Grimal, P 60
grotesque, the 58, 61, 97

Grundmann, C 82
Gutek,B 99

Hall, J 150
Hallam, J 52
Halloween costumes 59
hand-maiden 7, 24
handover 45
Hanson, J 164
Haque, O S 7, 160
hard physical work 23, 30, 48, 76
Hardacre, Cath 130–136, 160, 163
Hargreaves, R 72
Harran, M 115
Harris, N 118, 119
Harrison, T 139
Harter, S 8
Haswell, J 150
hauntings 83–85, 91
healers 34, 35, 39, 48
healing arts 36–39
healing spaces 82–83
health, nurses' own 24, 85; *see also*
    traumatic experiences whilst nursing
health care ethical standards 115
health care systems: business ethos of
    modern healthcare 29; cultural anxiety
    towards 161; mean/monstrous nurses
    within 108, 109, 110; mercy killings
    within 77; modern nursing deals with
    the abject 66; nurses who kill 77, 124,
    125; nursing's place in health care 19,
    52, 130–145; systemic dysfunction 68,
    130–145, 159
Hearn, M 51
Heberer, P 120
Hegge, M 38, 59
Hegney, D 152
Heidegger, M 135
Heinrich, K 30, 148
Helmstadter, C 2
hero-complexes 122
heroism 25, 155
Hewison, A 48
Hibbs, T 133
Hickey, E 121
hierarchies 21, 22, 30, 35
High Anxiety (Brooks, 1977) 99
higher degrees in nursing 36
highly skilled, nursing is 9, 10, 35,
    38, 106
history of nursing 2, 3–4, 30, 34–50,
    66, 146

Hochberg, M 101
Hochschild, A 27
holistic care 82, 149
Holmes, D 5, 66, 78, 117, 118, 125
Holocaust 114–121
home responsibilities 106, 135
Horner, A 88
horror genre 5, 83, 89, 91, 102, 137
Hospital Babylon (Edwards-Jones, 2011) 57
hospital dramas (TV) 17; *see also*
    TV dramas
Houlihan, Nurse Margaret "Hot Lips"
    53–54, 162
Houweling, L 58, 98
Howell, J 2
Hughes, S 91
humanisation 23, 51
humanistic philosophies 2
humiliation 58, 102, 151, 163
humility 36, 146, 148, 155
humour 23, 25–29, 52–53, 77; *see also*
    comedy
Humphrey, R 27
Hunter, K 104
Hurricane Katrina 75–77, 78
Hutchinson, M 109
Hutchinson, S 5
Huy, Q 28

I, Robot (Asimov, 1950) 153
I was there: Hurricane Katrina (The History
    Channel, 2015) 76
Iacono, M 55
Ibrahim, J 125
idealisation 23, 60
identity: diffusion 8, 123; evolution of
    identity 2; loss 133; nursing identity
    19; personal 26; professional identity
    7–8, 147
imagination 38, 39, 115
imposters 131, 132, 133
individualised care 42, 82, 140
infection control 21, 22
information source, nurses as patients' 46
innuendo 52, 54
Inside Amy Schumer (McFaul, 2014) 59
instrumentalism 135
integration 163
interdisciplinary analysis 6
intimate access to patients' bodies 5–6, 51,
    55, 65–66, 73, 74, 162
intimate connections between nurse and
    patient 74

intuition 38, 39, 40, 44, 90
Iris 60
Ironside (Young, 1967–1975) 17
irreverence 25
Ishikawa, Y 61

Jackson, D 5
James, S 153
Jan, C 141–142
Japan 61
Jeffrey, Betty 150
Jeffs, S 102
Jenkin, Pamela Rose 122
Jenner, C 38
job insecurity 5
Johns, C 38
Johnson, B 19, 21
Johnson, S 106
Jolley, R 122
Jones, A 91
Jones, Genene 122, 124
jouissance 18, 20–21
Jung, Carl 7, 115, 126, 142, 148,
    158, 159–160, 163, 164
justice, nursing as pursuit of 48, 121,
    126, 155

Kaiserswerth Deaconess Institute 98
Kakoudaki, D 53
Kalanithi, P 36
Kalisch, B 105, 158
Kalisch, P 105, 158
Karlsson, V 102
Kelly, D 91
Kelly, J 28
Kenny, Elizabeth 43–44
Kesey, K 103, 115
Kiefer, Nurse 116, 160, 164
kill, nurses who 4, 5, 114–129, 159
kindness 20, 23, 46, 72, 148
King, S (*Misery*) 99, 101–102, 115, 124,
    160, 161
King Arthur legend 148
Kissane, D 74
Knabb, R 75
Knight, S 6
knowledge: classifications of 37–38;
    embodied knowledge 90, 92; empirical
    knowledge 38, 41, 42, 46, 47, 92;
    ethical knowledge 40, 42; experiential
    knowledge 8, 35, 37, 42, 44, 46;
    feminine forms of 48; folk-wisdom 34,
    35; intuition 38, 39, 40, 44, 90;

mysterious 36–39; nurses as knowledge
workers 47; nursing knowledges in
action 44–48; nursing on the periphery
of 90–91; personal knowledge 38, 46;
scientific knowledge 37, 39, 41, 92,
109; and the scientific-technical
revolution 109; secret nature of nursing
knowledge 36; subjective knowledge
39; technical-rational knowledge 41,
47, 88, 92, 135, 162; used for bad/evil
purposes 101
Kondo, N 61
Kristeva, J 71–72, 89

Lacan, J 18
Ladd, C 87
Lagerwey, M 120
Lainz Angels of Death 122, 124
Lakeman, R 6
Lamb, M 5
Langton, R 55, 56
language issues 20, 43–44
Language of Kindness, The (Watson, 2018)
    36, 44–48, 85
Laredo, J 89
Last Offices 82
Lauder, W 143
Law and Order SVU (Wolf, 1999) 17
Lawler, J 6
lawsuits 123–124
laying out 19, 68, 73
Le Blanc, R 6
leadership 2, 52, 99, 151, 154
LeBlanc, R 158
legitimation of the profession 35, 42–43
Letter, Stephen 122
Levine, C G 8, 71
Life Magazine 60
life transitions, nurses practice at 155; *see*
    also death, dealing with; midwives
Lifton, R 118
liminal spaces 85–86, 137
Liminana-Gras, R 22
Lin, P 86
Lindsay, J 141
Lipsitz, G 124
litigation, fear of 123–124
"The Little Ship" 83
Litvak, A 84–85, 99
Locks, A 102
logical-rationalism 4
Loomis, R 148
López-Muñoz, F 138

Lorenza, G 90
lover, feminine archetype of 55–56, 60, 108
low pay 5, 110, 135, 162–163
low status 2, 19, 52, 106, 135, 162–163

M★A★S★H (Gelbart and Reynolds, 1972–1983) 53
Maben, J 106
MacKenzie, J 20
Macmillan, C 59, 61
MacWilliams, B 106
Magnolia (Anderson, 1999) 72–73, 75, 77–78, 162
maiden, archetypal 58
maim, nurses who 4
Maisel, Albert 138
male doctors 34, 35
male nurses 9, 21, 22, 34, 72–75, 97, 106, 123, 162
Mallett, R 17
managerialism 30, 82, 106, 124, 134
Manga, J 18
Manning, N 139
Manthorpe, J 139
manual labour, nursing seen as 109
marginalisation: ageing patients 20, 21; gender-based 30; in hospital systems 19; nurses work with the marginalised 5; of nursing 23, 30, 42–43, 59, 101
Margot, J 85
Markel, H 68
Marks, I 89
Martin, D 40
Martin Chuzzlewit (Dickens, 1853) 67–68, 69
masculinity 61, 101, 102, 106
MASH: A Novel About Three Army Doctors (Hooker, 1968) 53
mass murder 114–115, 119
matrons 21, 22, 52, 53, 100
McAllister, M 5, 6, 28, 30, 59, 71, 74, 85, 86, 88, 90, 117, 118, 125, 150, 151, 164
McCance, T 42
McCann, T 109
McCormack, B 42
McCrann, G 60
McEwan, Ian (*Atonement*) 1, 4, 9, 10, 18
McGowan, I W 85
McHugh, M 102, 134
McIntosh, B 135
McKinnon, C 57

media: and popular culture 10–13; popular culture and mass media 10–13; psychiatric care 139–142; questioning how nursing is portrayed in 107; shadow side of nursing 4; stories of "bad nursing" 3; unrealistic representations 3
medical murder 121–126
Medina, S 107
Meehan, John 108–109
memoirs 25–29, 36, 42, 44–48, 72, 75, 83–84, 85, 159
mental health nursing 26, 84, 85, 104–105, 107, 109, 136–142
mental health of nurses 77
mental illness 26, 27, 77, 116, 118, 136–142
mercy killings 5, 21, 77, 121, 122
Meskó, B 154
Meyers, J 124
middle management 22
middle-class profession, nursing becoming 2
Middleweek, B 124
midwives 34, 36, 118
Miles, L 72
military, nursing's links to 29, 53, 57, 60, 150
military-medical dramas 53
Mills, J 1
Misery (King 1987; Reiner, 1990) 99, 101–102, 115, 160, 161
mistakes 6, 10
Mitchell, David (*Cloud Atlas*) 59, 100–101
modelling, learning from 36
Molloy, L 6
monks 82
monstrous nurses 97–113
monstrous-feminine 97, 101, 102
Moore, K 124
moral codes 24, 25, 38
moral courage 48, 152
morale, staff 25, 53
Morgan, R 101
Morris-Thompson, T 36
mother figures 3, 55–56, 57, 60, 104, 108, 117
Mouton, M 115
Moyers, B 160
MRSA 21
Mullangi, S 36
multiple data sources, using 47
Mulvey, L 52

mundanity of nursing 19, 23, 148, 155
Muñoz, M 104, 105, 106
murdering nurses 114–129, 159
Murray, T 132
mysterious, nursing knowledge as 36–39

naïvity 53, 55, 58, 61
narrative medicine 36
National Health, The (Gold, 1973) 136
naughty nurse trope 51
Nazi nurses 5, 114–121, 126
near-death experiences 4
negative capability 6
Nelson, S 9, 46, 90, 97, 147
neo-liberalism 30, 91
Nichols, D 36, 43–44
Nicholson, H 99
Nietzsche, F 133, 134
Night Call Nurses (Kaplan, 1972) 57–58
night shifts 4, 66–67, 86, 89,
    90, 91
night terrors 85–87
Nightingale, Florence 1–2, 8, 30, 38,
    39, 68, 98
nihilism 133, 134, 135
Noakes, Nurse 100–101
"not knowing" 6
Nunan, D 149
nuns 29, 40, 82, 114, 150
Nun's Story, The (Hulme 1956;
    Zinnemann, 1959) 146, 155
Nurse (1981–1982) 98
Nurse (Anderson, 1979) 98
Nurse 3D (Aarniokoski, 2013) 58
Nurse Jackie (Brixius, Dunsky and Wallem,
    2009–2015) 23–25, 29, 30, 81, 131,
    135, 159, 160, 163
nurse-as-patient 139
nurse-as-sex-object metaphor 55–57, 59,
    60, 61; *see also* sexy nurse trope
Nurse's Story, A (Shalof, 2005) 36, 46–48
nursing identity 19
nursing neglect scandals 48
nurturing mother figures, nurses as 3,
    55–56, 57, 60
Nussbaum, M 55, 56
Nye, J 152

Oakley, J 99
oath 4
obedient, good nurses seen as 9, 10, 147
objectification of the nurse 55–57, 59, 61
objects of desire 51–64

O'Brien, C 36
O'Byrne, P 66
Oedipal ideas 56–57, 104, 108
Okie, S 76, 77
Oliviere, D 72
Ondaatje, M 147–148, 149
One Flew Over the Cuckoo's Nest (Forman,
    1975) 99, 103–108, 115, 160
O'Neill, C 3
Orr, D 30
otherness 104, 147
Outlander (Moore, 2014–current) 36–37
Overton, S 107
overweight nurses 20, 22, 100
Owens, M 85
Ozaras, G 34

pachinko parlours 61
pain killers 24
palliative care 35, 72, 73, 74, 87
Papantoniou, K 86
Paradise Road (Beresford, 1997) 150–152,
    155–156
paradoxes: abjection 68–69, 75; bad/evil
    nurses 97, 101; caring in society
    109–110; dealing with/fearing death
    90; ghosts 88; good nurse trope 10;
    Gothic 101–102; leaving/challenging
    the status quo 131, 133; monstrous
    nurses 101; *Nurse Jackie* (Brixius,
    Dunsky and Wallem, 2009–2015) 24;
    nurses who kill 125; popular culture
    sheds light on 161; of power 161;
    proper/improper 162; respect/fear of
    nursing knowledge 35, 130; sexual
    objectification of nurses 51, 55, 60, 61,
    62; slavery to a system 155; *Trust Me*
    (BBC, 2017) 132–133; value of nursing
    to society versus low pay/status 162
Parker, J 1
Parma, Nurse Phil 72–73, 77
parody 5
Parris, J 125
paternalism 3
pathways into nursing 25–26, 41
patience 27
patient satisfaction surveys 102–103
patient-nurse ratios 3, 102, 110
patient-nurse relationship 102; *see also*
    connections with patients; intimate
    access to patients' bodies
Patmore, C 9
patriarchy 97, 108

patronising attitudes 3, 52, 58, 100, 102
Patterson, J 73
Paul, E 150
Pearson, H 38
Peep Show (Redhead, 2004) 59
peer support 77, 86, 87, 151
Peplau, H E 2
Perez-Pena, R 123
Perron, A 66
personal knowledge 38, 46
person-centredness 2, 42, 82
Peterson, J 164
Petty, N 36
phallic imagery 53
physical work, nursing is hard 23, 30, 48, 76
Piatti-Farnell, L 75, 87, 91
podcasts 108, 122, 125
policies and bureaucracy: and the complexities of caring 91, 109; dehumanisation 110; depersonalisation 134; *Get Well Soon! My (Un)Brilliant Career as a Nurse* (Chambers, 2012) 28; managerialism 30, 82, 106, 124, 134; in Nazi Germany 117–118; neoliberal managerialism 30; *Nurse Jackie* (Brixius, Dunsky and Wallem, 2009–2015) 25; patronising attitudes 52; in transgressive texts 19, 20, 23; undermining ability to care 106
Polio 43
political correctness 19, 20–21, 52
Poovey, M 29
popular culture 10–13
pornography 5, 55, 57–59, 61
post-mortem care 82; *see also* laying out
Post-Traumatic Stress Disorder 77
Poulsen, J 132
poverty 65, 68, 135
power relations 51, 56, 59, 108, 133, 139, 152, 159–161, 164
practical "doers," nurses seen as 36
precise movement 38
Priebe, S 136
Proctor, R 117
profane-sacred, nursing rests between 37, 66, 71, 75
professional fulfillment 102
professional identity 7–8, 147
professionalisation of nursing 1, 35, 109, 117
projection 7, 73, 75, 160
propaganda 57, 60, 117, 119

protest actions 2–3, 110
psychiatric asylums 83–84, 103–108, 136–139, 140, 146
psychiatry 107
psychoanalytic feminism 98
psychodynamics 104
psychology, rise of 2
Psychoville (Lipsey, 2009-2011) 99
public health policy 22, 61, 118
purity tropes 58, 59

quality assurance standards 124

racial minorities 20
Rafter, N 136
Ratched (Netflix, proposed) 161
Ratched, Nurse 101, 103–108, 110, 115, 158, 164
reality TV 59
Redding, E 87
redemption 89, 150, 155
Redhead, Leigh 59
Reed, D 124
refugee camps 5
Reid, J 137
Reimer-Kirkham, S 81
religion, nursing's links to 29, 81–96, 98, 117–118, 119, 146
repression of own feelings *see* emotional labour
researcher-nurses 36
Resident, The (2018) 41
resilience 10, 47, 151–152
responsiveness 38
restitution narratives 6
Reverby, S 29, 66, 68
Richardson, N 102
rites of passage 70
rituals 4, 19, 82–83, 91
Roberts, S 7, 10, 98, 160
Robo Nurse (Usherwood, 2009) 153
robotic nurses 153–154, 156
Roenneberg, T 85
role models 8
romance novels 59
romanticisation 9, 23, 43, 161–162
Rook, H 92
Ross, P 43
routines 136–137, 140, 152, 154
Royle, N 88, 91
Rudge, T 5, 78
Rushmer, R 6

sacred in healthcare, role of the 81–96
sacred-profane, nursing rests in between
    37, 66, 71, 75
sadism 101
Saggurthi, S 6
Salzmann-Erikson, M 154
Samhain 36–37
sanctions, for failing to live up to
    stereotypes 9
Sandelowski, M 87, 154
Sanitarium (1998–current) 59
Sasso, L 110
Sawbridge, Y 48
Schott, C 8
Schulze, B 107
science fiction 152–153
scientific knowledge 37, 39, 41, 92, 109
Scott, S 139
Scrubbing In (Osper et al., 2013–current) 59
scrubs 58
Scrubs (2001–2010) 58
seaside postcards 52–53
second victim phenomenon 139, 152,
    163–164
secret nature of nursing knowledge 34–50
Sefton, Dan 132
Seinfeld (Cherones, 1989-1998) 55–57
self-acceptance 163
self-actualisation 149
self-awareness 150, 154–155
self-denial 1
selflessness 17, 19, 46, 54, 72, 101
self-preservation 21, 48
self-sacrifice 1, 2, 8
Seltzer, L 57
sensitivity 38–39, 47
sentimentalisation 10
serial killer nurses 5, 102, 121–126
sexism 51, 52, 56, 99, 106, 108, 162
sexualisation of nurses 51, 54, 55, 59,
    60, 108
sexy nurse trope 51, 52–57, 60, 61, 162
Seys, D 139, 152, 163
shadow side of nursing 4–7, 34–50, 115,
    126, 142, 158–163
Shafer, A 36
Shahsavari, H 28
Shalof, Tilda 36, 46–48
Sharp, S 106, 150
Sharpe, M 122, 125
Shields, L 5, 116, 120
shift work 135; *see also* night shifts
Shock (Werker, 1946) 99

shortages of nurses 5, 102, 108
Shutter Island (Scorsese, 2010) 99
Shuttleworth, A 22
Silveira, M 86
Simpson, P 123
Simpsons, The (Groening, 1989–current)
    17–18
"Sister" 82
Sister Kenny (Nichols, 1946) 36, 43–44
sitting with people, as key nursing role 45
60 Minutes (Harvey and Taylor, 1988)
    139, 140
skills of nursing 9, 10, 35, 38, 46, 47,
    102–103, 106, 117, 122, 123
Skyman, E 102
sleep, nurses own 86
Smith, A 60
Smith, D 51
Smith, K 87
Smith, S 5
Snake Pit, The (Ward 1946; Litvak, 1948)
    84–85, 99, 137–139, 140
Snelson, A 85
soap operas 17, 59
social activism 143, 155
social artefact, nursing as 2–3
Social Darwinism 117
social memory 5
socio-cultural phenomenon,
    nursing as 121
soft power 152
soldiers 53, 57, 60
solo working 90
Song a Day, A (Fleischer, 1936) 54, 55
sorcery 35
specialisations within nursing 109
spirituality 74–75, 81–96
Spooner, C 87
Stafford Hospital 131
Stanley, D 107
Stanley, N 139
starvation 120
stealing 24, 108, 163
Steffck 87
Steppe, H 117, 119, 121, 126
stereotypes: anti-nursing 107–108;
    based in the sacred aspects of nursing
    71; battleaxe 99; common 7; of
    femininity 161–162; mental health
    nursing 85; *Nurse Jackie* (Brixius,
    Dunsky and Wallem, 2009–2015) 23;
    nurses often defy 21; nursing identity 2,
    8–9, 158; pornography 58; reclaiming

and subverting 61; transgressions of 17, 19, 97; in TV dramas 17; virtue scripts 46; *see also* good nurse trope; sexy nurse trope
sterility 58
Stillwell, B 83–84
Stokowski, L 58
Storey, J 17
Storr, A 57
storytelling 6, 36, 52, 75, 83, 87–88, 91, 92, 122, 158
Stratiev, S 53
Street, A 74
strength of mind 47
strengths of nurses 48
stressful nature of work 5, 7, 77, 86, 160
strike action 2–3, 110
student nurses 24, 28
subjective knowledge 39
subjective/objective dialectic 35, 39
sublimation 75
subversiveness 4–5, 17, 21
suffering, moving towards 38, 41, 48
Sullivan, E 106
Summers, H 55, 158
Summers, S 55, 158
supernatural occurrences 86, 90
superstitions 85–87
surface acting 27
Svedlund, M 102–103
Svoboda, R 3
swearing 24, 26

T4 policy 117–119
taboo 5, 6, 23, 56, 72, 90
Tahghighi, M 86
Tallis, Nurse Briony (*Atonement*) 1, 2, 3, 9–10, 18, 60
Tarrant, J 126
Taylor, J 71
team work 45, 151, 155
technical-rational knowledge 41, 47, 88, 92, 135, 162
technological advances in nursing 153–154
Templeton, S 106
Thakur, M 6
Thalidomide 40
therapeutic communities 139–142
thinking versus doing 35–36
Timbrell, J 6
Tinker, R 122
Tomlinson, D 136

"too posh to wash" 109
totalitarian institutions 107
Townsville Hospital, Queensland 139–142
toxic workplaces 164
training: dehumanisation 28; focus on caring and cleanliness 68–69; *Get Well Soon! My (Un)Brilliant Career as a Nurse* (Chambers, 2012) 26; history of nursing 2; and the modern health care system 131; professional levels of 106, 109; secret nature of nursing knowledge 36
transgender people 17
transgressive texts 17–33, 37
translocated ideal 104
traumatic backgrounds (nurses') 27, 124–125, 147–148
traumatic experiences whilst nursing 77, 89, 91, 107, 138–139, 147–149, 151, 163–164
Traynor, M 5, 146
triage 76
Trinkoff, A 110
true crime 108–109, 122, 124, 125
Trust Me (BBC, 2017) 130–136, 142, 160, 163
Truth About Nursing 4, 107
turnover rate in nursing profession 5
TV dramas 17, 36–39, 40–42, 53, 58–59, 98, 108, 125, 130–136, 159, 161; *see also specific dramas*
Tyler, T R 8

uncanny 91
unconscious 7, 89, 90, 115, 160, 164
understaffing 140; *see also* shortages of nurses
unethical practices 5
uniforms 28–29, 51, 52, 54, 58–59, 61, 140
unsettled/unsettling stories 88–90
unsociable hours 162–163
Usherwood, F 153, 154

value of nursing, nurses knowing 154–155
values 1, 2, 10, 55, 119, 120, 121, 133, 134
Vicinus, M 8
video games 59
violence 7, 22–23, 139, 146, 160
virtue 164

virtue scripts 46
visibility 36
vocation/calling, nursing as a 25, 82, 146, 147
Vogus, T 125
Vronsky, P 121
vulnerability 89, 122, 142–143, 159, 160

Wadsworth, P 6
Wainright, P 38
Wallaston, S 132
Walton, Henrietta 76
Wang, R 153
War Nurse (1930) 69–70
Ward, Mary Jane 137
Ward, The (Carpenter, 2010) 99, 161
Ward 10B, Townsville Hospital, Queensland 139–142
wartime 5, 9, 60, 69–70, 114, 117, 147–148, 150, 155
Watson, Christie 36, 41, 44–48, 85
Watts, A 163
Waytz, A 7, 160
Weatherhead, R 140
Welsford, E 56
whistleblowing 131, 135, 142
White, J 38
White Coolies (Jeffrey, 1954) 150
white uniforms 29, 58–59, 61, 116, 140
Whitman, Walt 70
Wicks, D 36
Wiese, M 90
Wilde, Nurse Kim 19, 163

Wilkes, Nurse Annie 101–102, 115
Willis, P 11
Wilson, D 121–122
Wilson, E 140, 141
Wippermann, W 119
witchcraft 34–35
Wolf, S 126
Wolf, Z 6, 158
Wolff, T 56
Woolf, Virginia 89–90
working classes 22, 24, 35, 109, 135, 162–163
World Health Organization 142
world views 46
Worth, J 40
"The Wound Dresser" (Whitman, 1897) 70
wounded healer archetype 148–150, 156, 160
Wright, D 90
Wright, J 1

Yardley, E 121–122
Yashinsky, D 91, 92
Yolken, E 118
Yorker, B 123
Young Doctors, The (1976-1983) 59, 99

Zalla, C 17
Zizek, S 18, 88
Zlosnik, S 88
Zweig, C 126

Printed in the United States
by Baker & Taylor Publisher Services